THEORY & PRACTICAL A

EKG TEXTBOOK

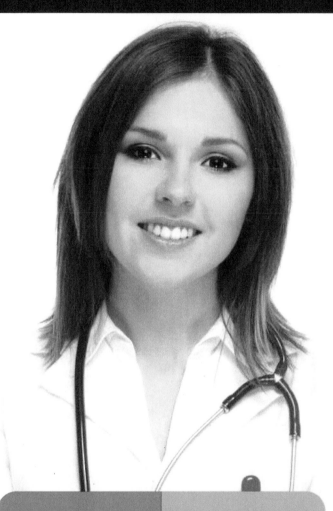

STUDENT
RESOURCES

INSTRUCTOR
RESOURCES

www.mcgilleducation.com

E-LEARNING

OTHER BOOKS

AUTHOR: SULTAN KHAN   FAISAL FAROOQ, MD

McGill Education Series: EKG TEXTBOOK

THEORY & PRACTICAL APPROACH
EKG TEXTBOOK

2nd Edition

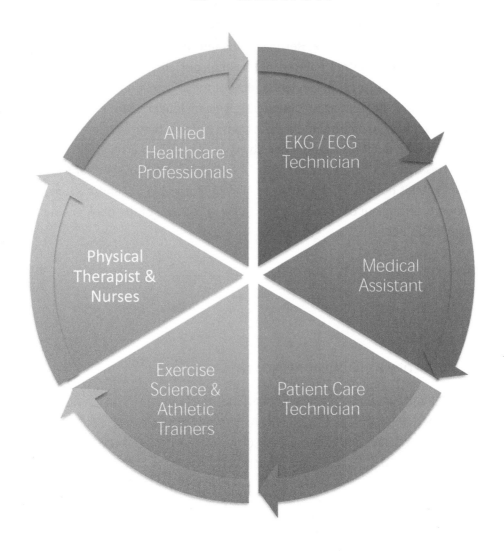

Allied Healthcare Professionals

EKG / ECG Technician

Medical Assistant

Patient Care Technician

Exercise Science & Athletic Trainers

Physical Therapist & Nurses

SULTAN KHAN **FAISAL FAROOQ, MD**

NATIONAL CERTIFICATION PREPARATION BOOK

NOTICE:

Knowledge and practice in this field are constantly changing, the publisher has the right to update, modify or change the content of this book at any time. Publisher cautions that this publication is not intended as a substitute for professional judgment of trained medical personnel, in other words this book is not intended to be a substitute for medical advice, treatment, evaluation or diagnosis. Seek medical advice from a qualified healthcare professional in context to a medical condition. Never ignore a medical advice as a result of information found or read in this book. Relying on the information in the book is solely at your own risk. Publisher, author, editors, advisors of this book disclaims all liability for any inaccuracies, omission, misuse, or misunderstanding of the information contained in this book. It is the responsibility of the treating practitioner, relying on independent expertise and knowledge of the patient, to determine the best treatment and method of application for the patient. The author and publisher assume no liability for any kind of errors or omissions of information in this book. To the full extent of the law, neither the publisher nor the author, editors, advisors of this book will not assume any liability for any injury and/or damage to person or property arising out of or related to any use or reliance of the book in whole or in part contained in this book.

BY

AUTHORS

PREFACE

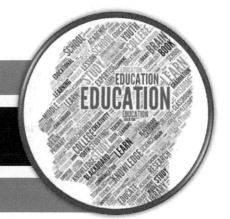

The book has been written and structured to simplify the process of learning concepts in EKG.

In our career of teaching EKG, numerous students have shown a lack of understanding when it comes to the concept of EKG, Our aim is to make the process of learning easy for students.

The book covers most of the essential topics required to understand the concepts of EKG, it is concise and to the point. As per our experience we believe that "Learning process can only be easy when the contents for learning are laid out in a simplified manner."

Thus we have separated the contents of the book as follows:

| EKG Anatomy & Physiology | EKG Theory | EKG Clinical | EKG Competency |

The book contains different case scenarios and various types of EKG's

(12 Lead EKG, 15 Lead EKG Adult & Pediatrics, 5 Lead EKG, 3 Lead EKG, Stress Testing and more)

Easy to understand graph interpretations in tabular format.

Understanding the EKG concept can be difficult at times, an initiative has been taken to make EKG simple and easy to learn, I hope our written work will help students.

Congratulations on choosing a healthcare career.

We would like to thank our beautiful families for their support, as this project may not have been possible without their support.

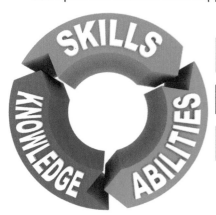

BY AUTHOR

CHAPTER 1 ANATOMY & PHYSIOLOGY

CHAPTER 2 EKG THEORY

CHAPTER 4 EKG CLINICAL COMPETENCY

CHAPTER 5 EKG CERTIFICATION EXAM REVIEW

STUDY MODULES

MODULE 1 : ANATOMY & PHYSIOLOGY

MODULE 2 : EKG THEORY

MODULE 3 : EKG CLINICAL

MODULE 4 : EKG CLINICAL COMPETENCY

MODULE 5 : EKG PRACTICE EXAM 100 QUESTIONS

CHAPTER 1

ANATOMY AND PHYSIOLOGY

ANATOMY & PHYSIOLOGY OF THE HEART

The Heart is a muscular organ that pumps the blood throughout the circulatory system. It is situated in the mediastinum. The boundaries of the mediastinum are:

- **Superiorly** (thoracic inlet)
- **Inferiorly** (diaphragm)
- **Anteriorly** (sternum, manubrium & costal cartilages)
- **Posteriorly** (bodies of thoracic vertebrae)
- **Laterally** (mediastinal pleura)

The Heart is made up of four chambers, two atria and two ventricles. The musculature of the ventricles is thicker than that of atria. The musculature of the left ventricle is thicker than that of the right ventricle. Force of contraction of the heart depends on the muscle size.

RIGHT SIDE OF THE HEART

Right side of the heart has two chambers, **right atrium** and **right ventricle.** The right atrium is a thin walled and low pressure chamber. It consists of the pacemaker known as **sino-atrial node** that produces cardiac impulses and **atrio-ventricular node** which is present at the boundaries between the atria and ventricles that conducts the impulses to the ventricles.

The right atrium receives venous **(deoxygenated)** blood via two large veins:

1. **Superior vena cava** that returns venous blood from the head, neck and upper limbs
2. **Inferior vena cava** that returns venous blood from lower parts of the body

The right atrium communicates with the right ventricle through the tricuspid valve. The wall of the right ventricle is thick. Venous blood from the right atrium enters the right ventricle through the opening of tricuspid valve. From the right ventricle, **pulmonary artery** arises. It carries the venous blood from right ventricle to the lungs. In the lungs, the deoxygenated blood is oxygenated. This is an exception in the human body where an artery is carrying venous blood.

LEFT SIDE OF THE HEART

The left side of the heart has two chambers, the **left atrium** and the **left ventricle.** The left atrium is a thin walled and low pressure chamber. It receives oxygenated blood from the lungs through pulmonary veins. This is an exception in the human body, where a vein is carrying oxygenated blood. Blood from left atrium enters the left ventricle through the mitral valve (bicuspid valve). The wall of the left ventricle is very thick. The left ventricle pumps the oxygenated blood to different parts of the body through the aorta.

Points to remember: *Arteries carry oxygenated blood and veins carry deoxygenated blood, exceptions are pulmonary artery and pulmonary vein.* ***(Pulmonary Artery carries deoxygenated blood) (Pulmonary Vein carries oxygenated blood)***

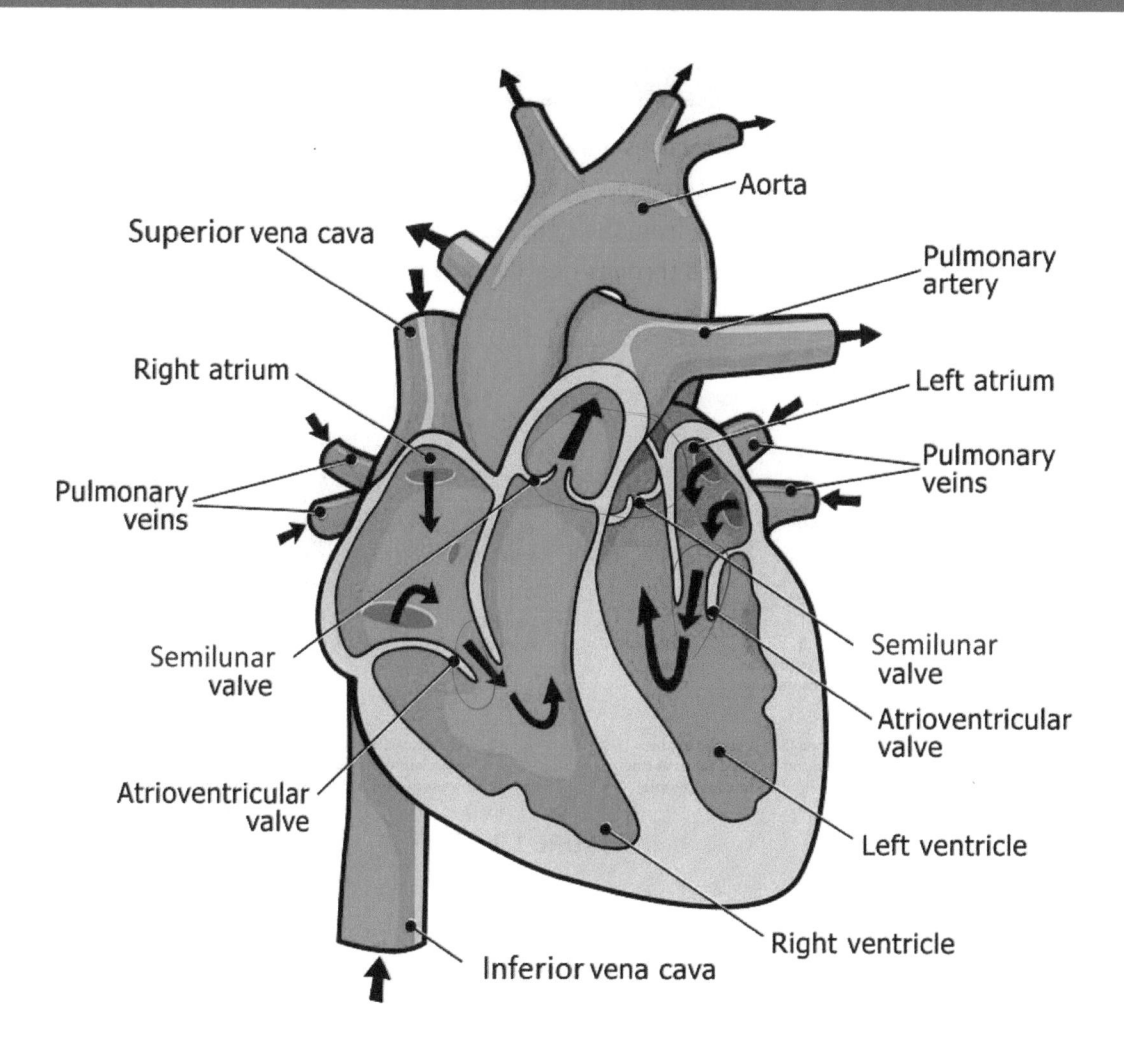

FIGURE 1.1

TABLE 1.1

	RIGHT	LEFT
UPPER CHAMBERS	**ATRIUM** Receives deoxygenated blood from superior and inferior vena cava.	**ATRIUM** Receives oxygenated blood from both (right and left) lungs via the pulmonary vein.
LOWER CHAMBERS	**VENTRICLE** Receives the deoxygenated blood from right atrium via the tricuspid valve and pumps it out of the heart via the pulmonary artery to the right and the left lung.	**VENTRICLE** Receives oxygenated blood from left atrium via the bicuspid valve and pumps it out of the heart to the rest of the body via the aorta.

VALVES OF THE HEART

There are four valves in human heart. Two valves are in between atria and the ventricles called atrioventricular valves. Other two are the semilunar valves, placed at the opening of blood vessels arising from ventricles, namely pulmonary artery arising from the right ventricle and aorta arising from the left ventricle. Valves of the heart permit the flow of blood through heart in only one direction.

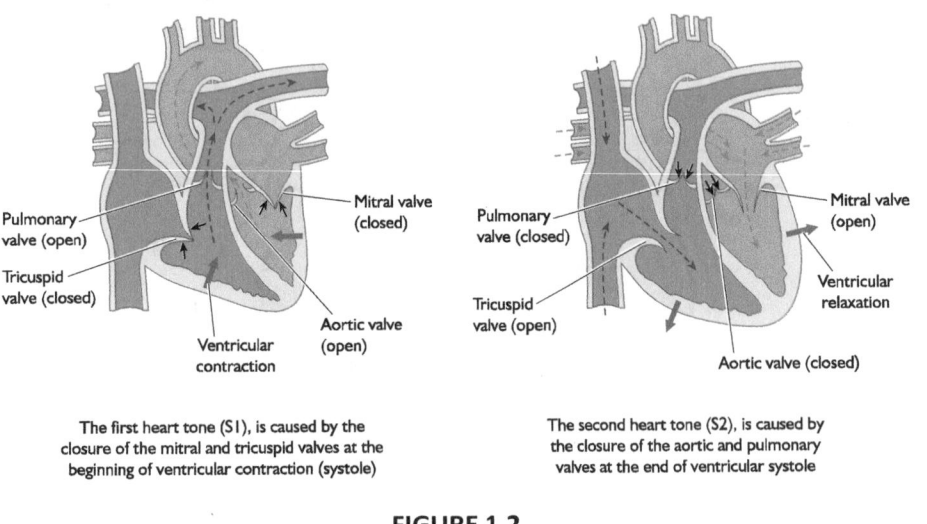

The first heart tone (S1), is caused by the closure of the mitral and tricuspid valves at the beginning of ventricular contraction (systole)

The second heart tone (S2), is caused by the closure of the aortic and pulmonary valves at the end of ventricular systole

FIGURE 1.2

Atrioventricular Valves

The right atrioventricular valve is known as the **tricuspid valve** and it is formed by three cusps. The left atrioventricular valve is called **mitral valve** or **bicuspid valve.** It is formed by two valvular **cusps** or flaps. The brim of the atrioventricular valves is attached to atrioventricular ring, which is the fibrous connection between the atria and ventricles. Cusps of the valves are attached to **papillary muscles** by means of the **chordate tendineae.** Papillary muscles arise from inner surface of the ventricles. Papillary muscles play an important role in the closure of the cusps and in preventing the back flow of blood from the ventricle into the atria during ventricular contraction. Atrioventricular valves open only towards the ventricles and prevent the backflow of blood into the atria.

Semilunar Valves

Semilunar valves are present at the openings of the pulmonary artery and the systemic aorta and are known as **pulmonary valve** and **aortic valve** respectively. Because of the half moon shape, these two valves are called semilunar valves. Semilunar valves are made up of three flaps. Semilunar valves open only towards the pulmonary artery and aorta thereby preventing the backflow of blood into the ventricles.

Points to remember: *The main function of the valve is to prevent the backflow, valves found in the heart is to prevent the backflow of blood within the chamber.*

SEPTA OF THE HEART

The right and left atria are separated from one another by a fibrous septum called **inter-atrial septum.** The

right and left ventricle are separated from one another by **inter-ventricular septum.** The upper part of this

septum is a membranous structure, whereas the lower part of it is muscular in structure.

The pathway of blood flow through the heart

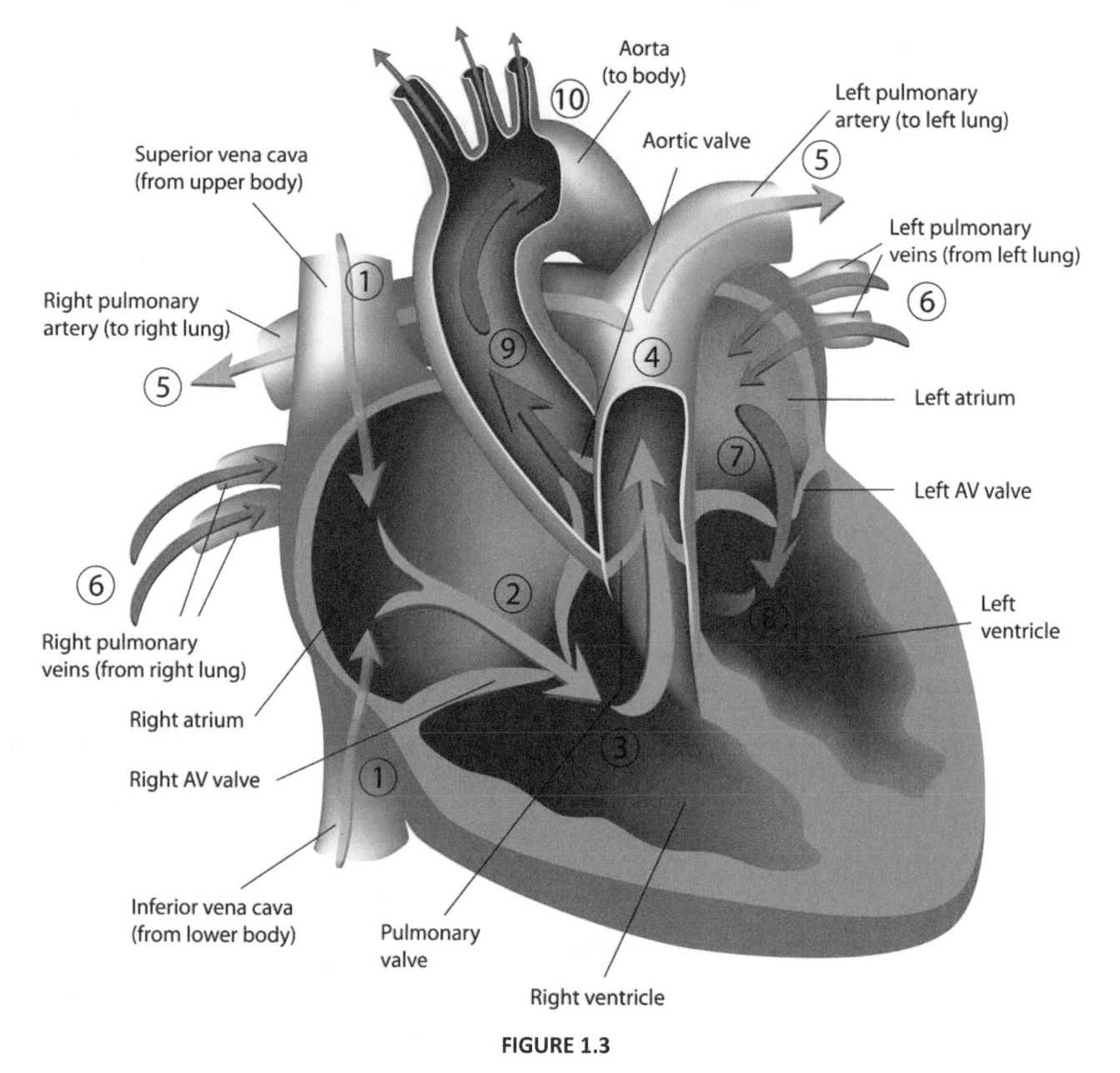

FIGURE 1.3

Flow of blood through the heart

Chapter 1: ANATOMY & PHYSIOLOGY

CIRCULATION OF BLOOD THROUGH THE HEART

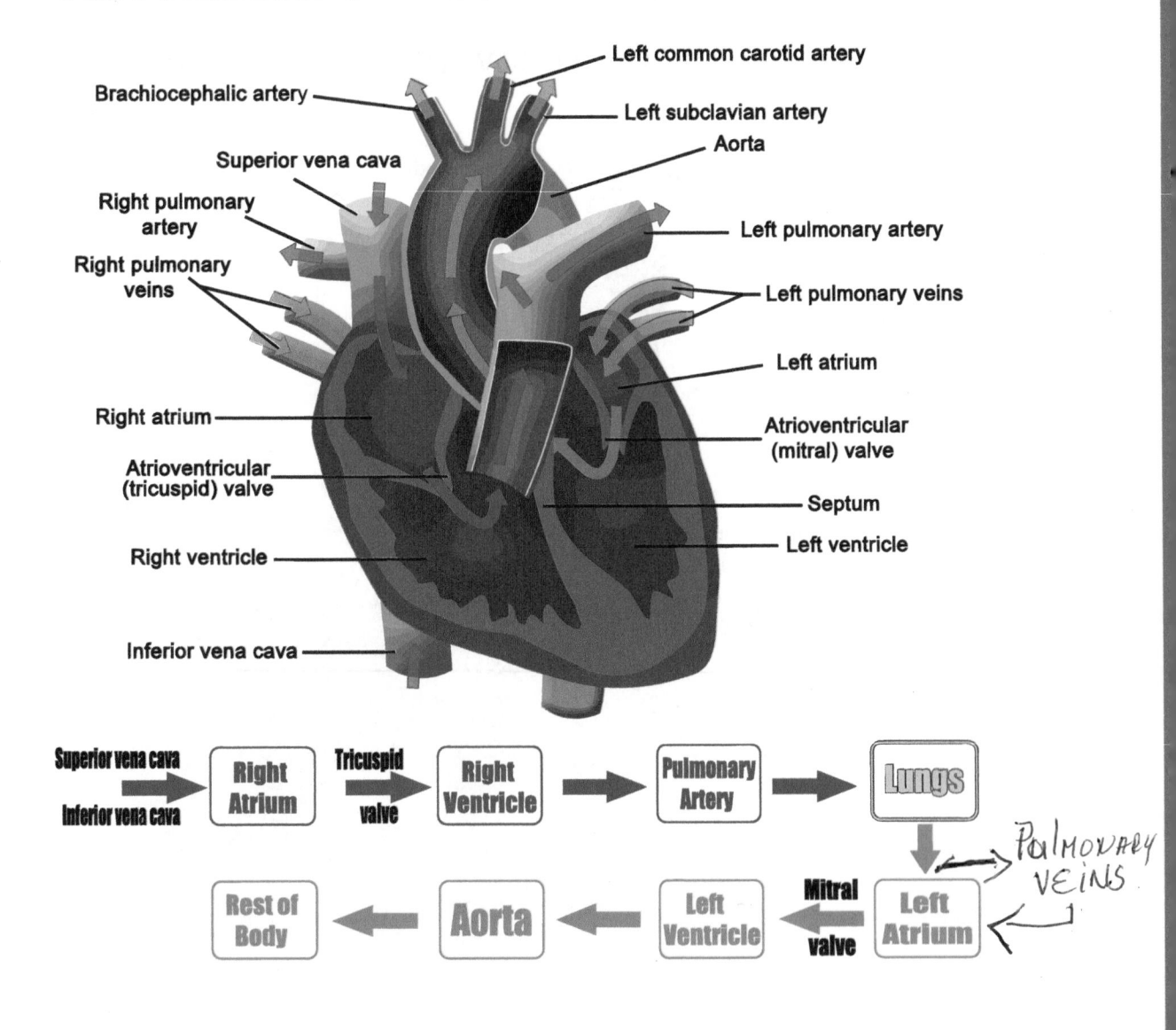

FIGURE 1.4

Summary of blood flow from superior and inferior vena cava to the rest of the body

LAYERS OF THE HEART

The Heart is made up of three layers of tissues:

1. **Outer Pericardium** - is the outermost layer of the heart covering the heart externally.

2. **Middle Myocardium** - is the main muscular layer forming the atria and ventricles. This layer also contains blood vessels and nerves.

3. **Inner Endocardium** - is the innermost layer of the heart.

WHAT IS PERICARDIUM?

The pericardium is a thin double-layered sac which encloses and covers the heart. The layers of the pericardium consist of:

- **Fibrous Pericardium (FP)** - outermost layer
- **Serous Pericardium (SP)** - lies on the inner surface of the fibrous pericardium

  The serous pericardium is further divided into two layers

  o Parietal layer of the serous pericardium (Parietal Pericardium)

  o Visceral layer of the serous pericardium (Visceral Pericardium)

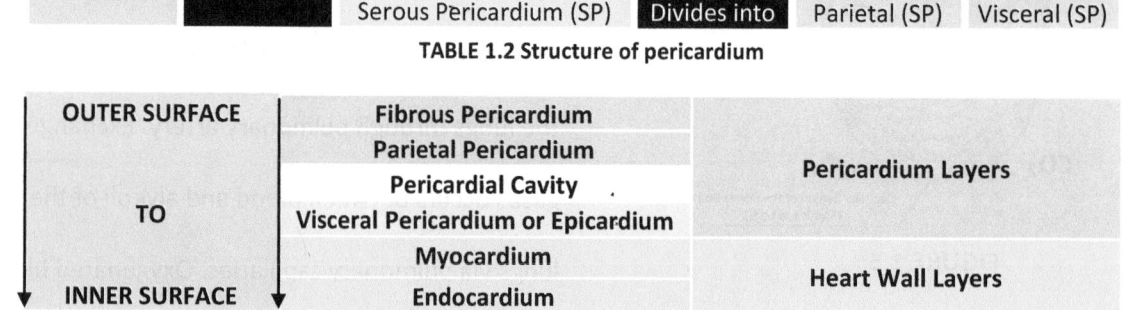

Pericardium	Divides into	Fibrous Pericardium (FP)	No further divisions		
		Serous Pericardium (SP)	Divides into	Parietal (SP)	Visceral (SP)

TABLE 1.2 Structure of pericardium

OUTER SURFACE	Fibrous Pericardium	Pericardium Layers	
	Parietal Pericardium		
TO	Pericardial Cavity		
	Visceral Pericardium or Epicardium		
	Myocardium	Heart Wall Layers	
INNER SURFACE	Endocardium		

TABLE 1.3 Layers of pericardium and heart

The space between the two layers of the serous pericardium consists of the pericardial space or pericardial cavity which contains the pericardial fluid. Pericardial fluid is an ultra filtrate of plasma, acting as a lubricant between the visceral and parietal layer of the pericardium. Fluid is contained within the layers of pericardium that constantly lubricates the rubbing surfaces thereby reducing the friction between the layers.

DIVISIONS OF CIRCULATION

Blood flows through two divisions of the circulatory system:

1. Systemic Circulation

2. Pulmonary Circulation

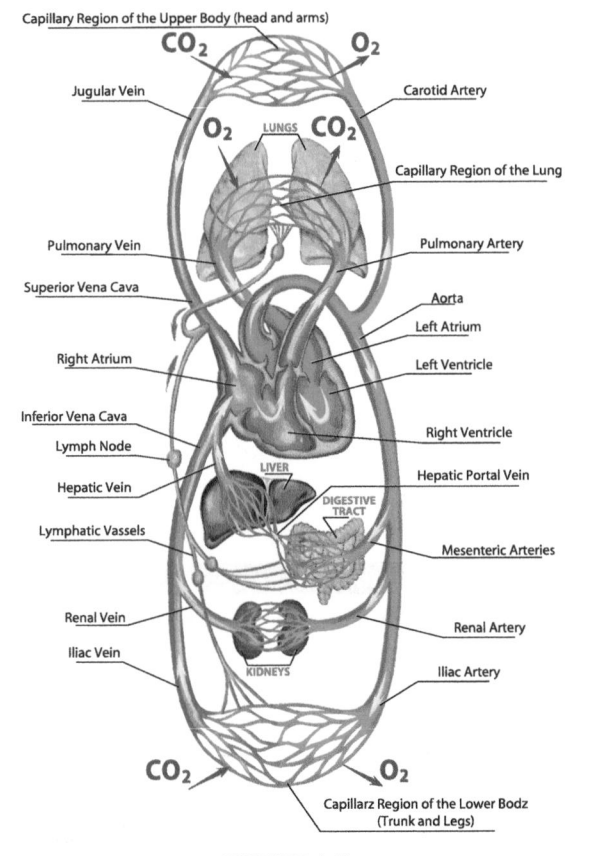

FIGURE 1.5

SYSTEMIC CIRCULATION

Systemic circulation is otherwise known as **greater circulation**. Blood pumped from the left ventricle passes through a series of blood vessels, from artery to arteriole system and reaches the tissues via the capillaries. Exchange of various substances between blood and the tissues occur at the capillaries. After exchange of materials, blood enters the venules and then the vein and eventually returns to right atrium of the heart *(via the superior and inferior vena cava)*. From the right atrium, blood enters the right ventricle. Thus, through systemic circulation, oxygenated blood is supplied from the heart to the tissues and the venous blood returns to the heart from the tissues.

HEART ➜ TISSUE

TISSUE ➜ HEART

PULMONARY CIRCULATION

Pulmonary circulation is otherwise called **lesser circulation.** Blood is pumped from right ventricle to the lungs through pulmonary artery. Exchange of gases occurs between blood and alveoli of the lungs via pulmonary capillaries. Oxygenated blood returns to left atrium through the pulmonary veins. Thus, left side of the heart contains oxygenated or arterial blood and the right side of the heart contains deoxygenated or venous blood.

Diastole & Systole
of
Human Heart

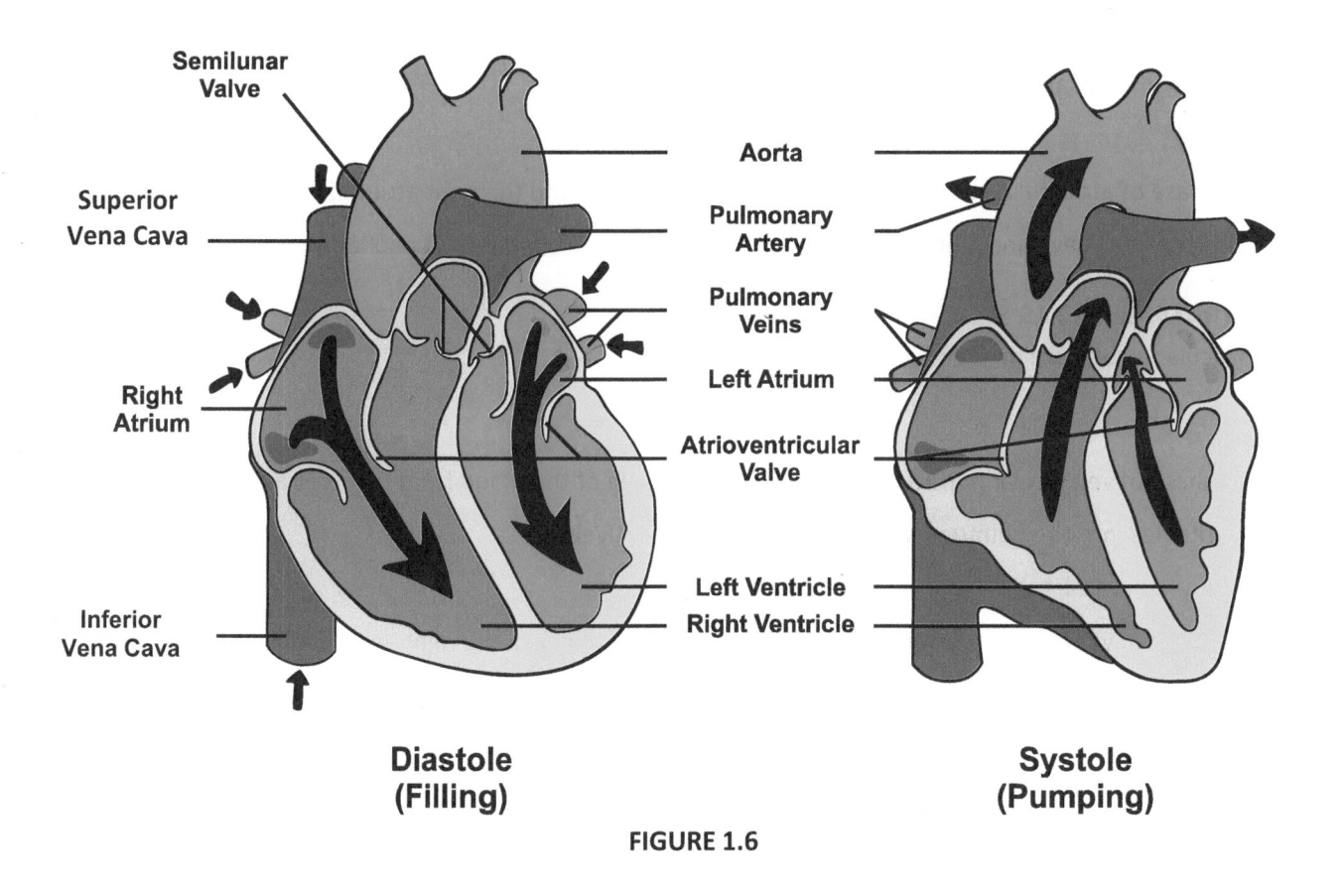

Diastole
(Filling)

Systole
(Pumping)

FIGURE 1.6

Cardiac cycle is defined as a sequence of **coordinated events** taking place in the heart during each

heartbeat. Each heartbeat consists of two major phases called **systole** and **diastole**. During ventricular

diastole, heart relaxes and blood from the right atrium is filled into the right ventricle by opening of

tricuspid valve and blood from the left atrium is filled into the left ventricle by opening of the bicuspid or

mitral valve simultaneously. During ventricular systole, ventricles contract and pumps the blood from

the right ventricle into the pulmonary artery with closure of the tricuspid valve and opening of the

pulmonary valve and from the left ventricle into the aorta with closure of the bicuspid or mitral valve and

opening of aortic valve. All these changes are repeated during every heartbeat, in a cyclic manner.

Chapter 1: ANATOMY & PHYSIOLOGY

DIVISIONS OF CARDIAC CYCLE

ATRIAL EVENTS

Atrial events are divided into two divisions:

1. **Atrial Systole**

   A phase of atrial contraction resulting in the pumping of the blood from the right atrium into the right ventricle, and from the left atrium into the left ventricle.

2. **Atrial Diastole**

   A phase of atrial relaxation resulting in the filling of blood into the right atrium from superior and inferior vena cava and filling of blood into the left atrium from the right and left pulmonary veins.

VENTRICULAR EVENTS

Ventricular events are divided into two divisions:

1. **Ventricular Systole**

   A phase of ventricular contraction resulting in pumping of the blood from the right and left ventricles into the pulmonary artery and aorta respectively.

2. **Ventricular Diastole**

   A phase of ventricular relaxation resulting in filling of blood into the right ventricle from the right atrium and filling of blood into the left ventricle from the left atrium.

Blood Flow through the body

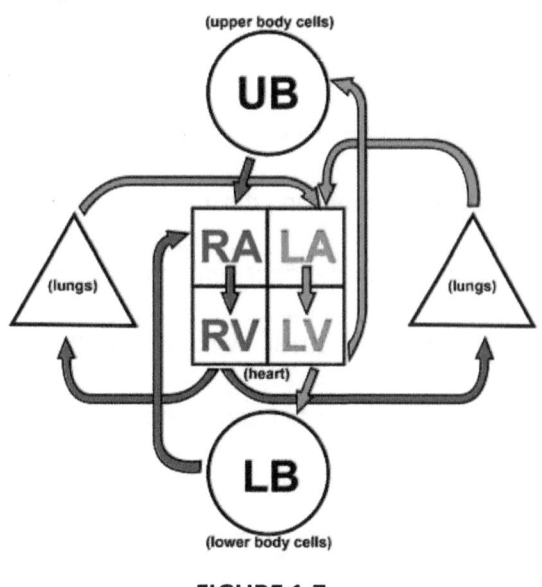

FIGURE 1.7

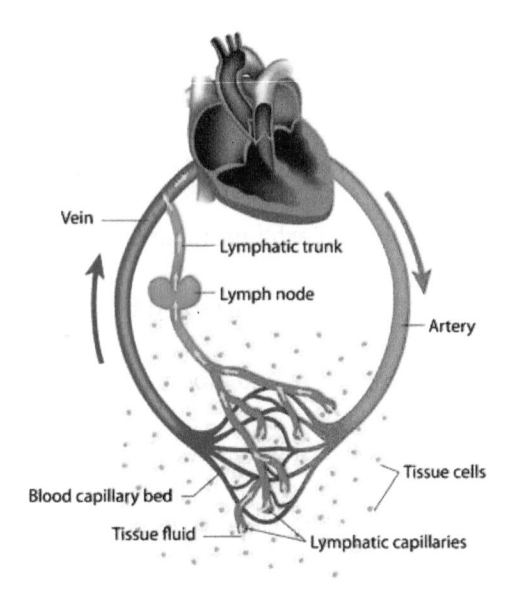

FIGURE 1.7a

Chapter 1: ANATOMY & PHYSIOLOGY

CARDIAC OUTPUT

Cardiac output is the amount of blood pumped from each ventricle. Usually, it refers to left ventricular output through aorta. Cardiac output is the most important factor in cardiovascular system, because rate of blood flow through different parts of the body depends on the cardiac output.

STROKE VOLUME
Stroke volume is the amount of blood pumped out by each ventricle during each beat.

HEART RATE
Number of times the heart beats in one minute.

CARDIAC OUTPUT
Cardiac output is the amount of blood pumped out by each ventricle in one minute. It is the product of stroke volume and heart rate.

- Increase cardiac output may indicate high circulatory volume

- Decrease cardiac output may indicate low circulatory volume or decrease in the strength of ventricular contraction.

Cardiac Output (CO) = Stroke Volume (SV) × Heart Rate (HR)

CO (ml/min) = SV (ml/beat) x HR (bpm)

ml/min: milliliters of blood per minute

ml/beat: milliliters of blood per beat

bpm: beats per minute

For example: a person with heart rate of 74 and stroke volume of 70 will have a cardiac output of 5180ml/min. (SV 70ml/beat X HR 74bpm = CO 5180ml/min)

CARDIAC INDEX

Cardiac index is the minute volume expressed in relation to square meter of body surface area. It is defined as the amount of blood pumped out per ventricle/minute/square meter of the body surface area.

Cardiac Index = Cardiac Output / Body Surface Area.

EFFECT OF NERVOUS SYSTEM ON HEART

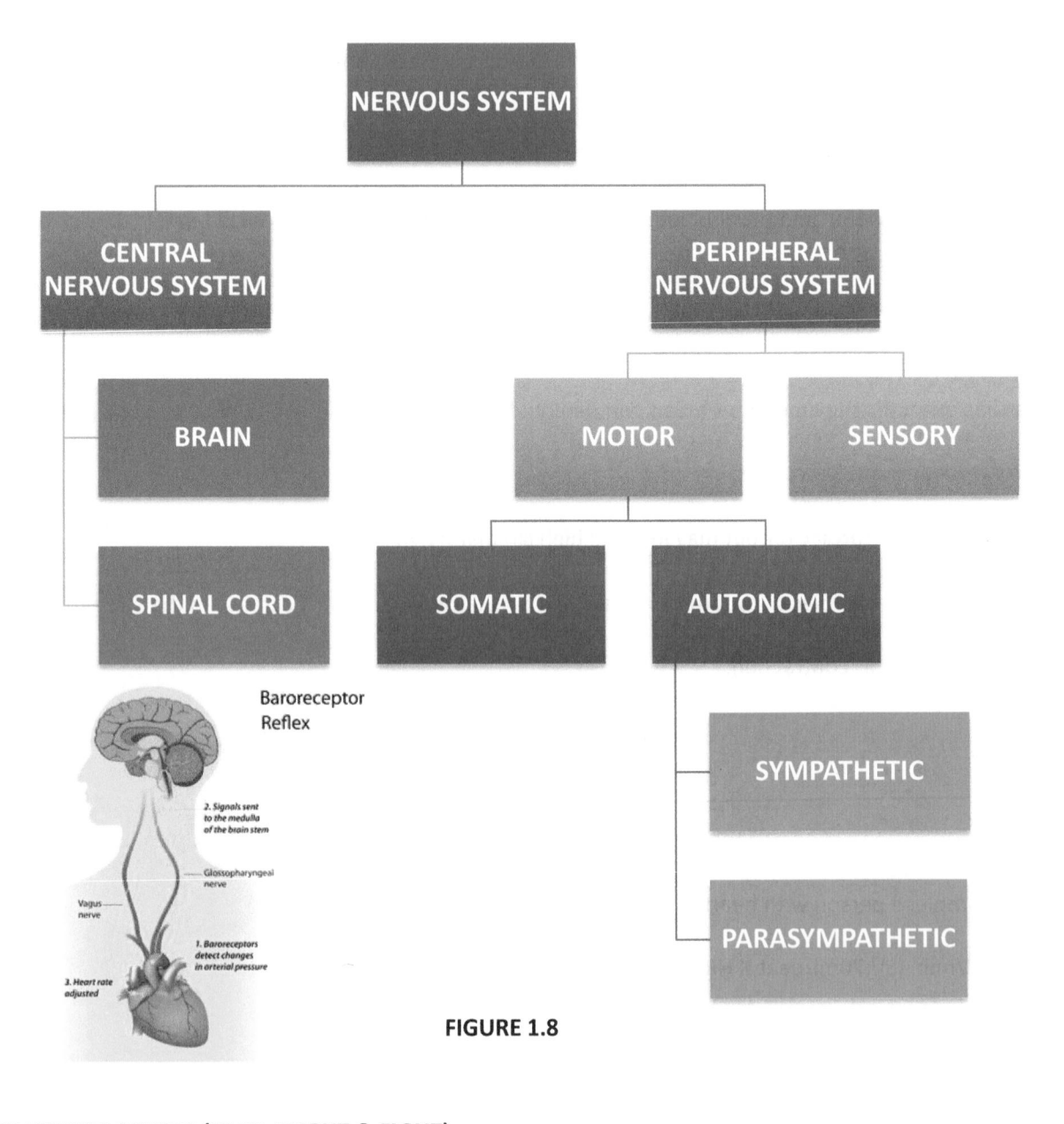

FIGURE 1.8

SYMPATHETIC CAUSES (FEAR, FLIGHT & FIGHT)

INCREASE HEART RATE → INCREASE STROKE VOLUME → INCREASE CARDIAC OUTPUT

PARASYMPATHETIC CAUSES

DECREASE HEART RATE → DECREASE STROKE VOLUME → NORMAL CARDIAC OUTPUT

FIGURE 1.9

The Cardiac Conduction System

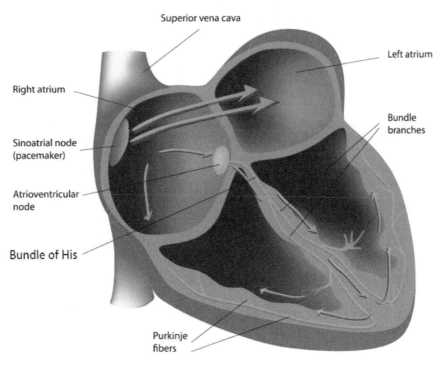

FIGURE 1.10

Pacemaker

Natural Pacemaker is the structure of heart from which the impulses for heartbeats are produced.

It is formed by the pacemaker cells called "**P**" cells.

1. *Sino-Atrial Node (SA Node)*
2. *Inter-Nodal Fibers*
3. *Atrio-Ventricular Node (AV Node)*
4. *Bundle of His*
5. *Purkinje Fibers*

Autonomic nervous system plays a vital role in regulating cardiac output. Pacemakers are innervated by autonomic nervous system. Intensity of ventricular contraction depends on the initial stretching of the cardiac tissues, frank-starling law explains that the increased volume of blood within the ventricle during the diastole will cause an increase in the intensity of the stretches within the ventricular wall of the heart, causing the cardiac muscles of the ventricle to contract more forcefully.

Points to remember: The intensity of final contraction is the resultant of the initial stretch force, higher intensity stretching of the tissue within the normal limits will lead to a higher intensity contraction of the tissue.

Chapter 1: ANATOMY & PHYSIOLOGY

Understanding Polarization

When cardiac cells are at rest and no activity is taking place, the ion concentration is at the resting potential.

Understanding Depolarization

When an impulse is generated in the heart the ion starts crossing the cell membranes causing the action potential to start with a rapid depolarization. The movement of ions across the cell membrane leads to a contraction of the cardiac muscles. Depolarization occurs because of **INFLUX** of more calcium ions. Unlike in other tissues, the depolarization in SA node is mainly due to the influx of calcium ions, rather than sodium ions. This event leads to the contraction of the cardiac muscles.

Understanding Repolarization

After rapid depolarization, repolarization starts. It is due to the **EFFLUX** of potassium ions from the pacemaker fibers. Potassium channels remain open for a longer time, causing **EFFLUX** of more potassium ions. It leads to the development of more negativity, beyond the level of resting membrane potential. It exists only for a short period. This event leads to the relaxation of the cardiac muscle with the ions returning to a resting state.

There are three types of internodal fibers that connect the Sino-Atrial Node (SA Node) & Atrio-Ventricular Node (AV NODE):

1. Anterior Internodal Fibers of Bachman

2. Middle Internodal Fibers of Wenckebach

3. Posterior Internodal Fibers of Thorel

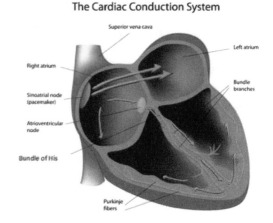

The Cardiac Conduction System

Chapter 1: ANATOMY & PHYSIOLOGY

CORONARY ARTERIES

Coronary arteries supply blood to the heart muscles, namely right and left coronary arteries, which are

the first branches of aorta.

Right and Left Coronary Arteries

Right coronary artery supplies whole of the right ventricle and posterior portion of left ventricle.

Left coronary artery supplies mainly the anterior and lateral parts of left ventricle. There are many

variations in diameter of coronary arteries.

Right Coronary Artery

The right coronary artery branches into:

- Right Marginal Artery (RMA)
- Posterior Descending Artery (PDA)

Left Coronary Artery

The left main coronary artery branches into:

- Circumflex Artery
- Left Anterior Descending Artery (LAD)
- Oblique Marginal Artery
- Diagonal Artery

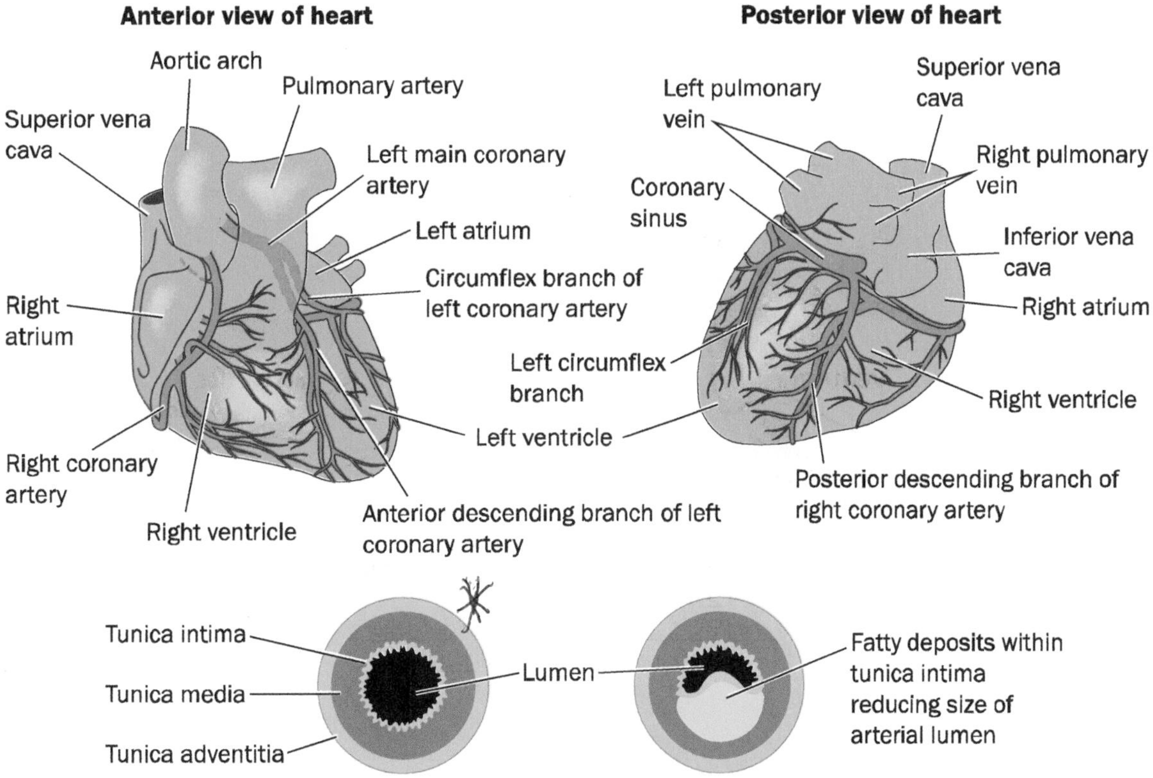

Anterior view of heart

Aortic arch
Pulmonary artery
Superior vena cava
Left main coronary artery
Left atrium
Circumflex branch of left coronary artery
Right atrium
Right coronary artery
Right ventricle
Anterior descending branch of left coronary artery
Left ventricle

Posterior view of heart

Left pulmonary vein
Superior vena cava
Coronary sinus
Right pulmonary vein
Inferior vena cava
Right atrium
Left circumflex branch
Right ventricle
Posterior descending branch of right coronary artery

Tunica intima
Tunica media
Tunica adventitia
Lumen
Fatty deposits within tunica intima reducing size of arterial lumen

FIGURE 1.11

Chapter 1: ANATOMY & PHYSIOLOGY

Artery & Vein

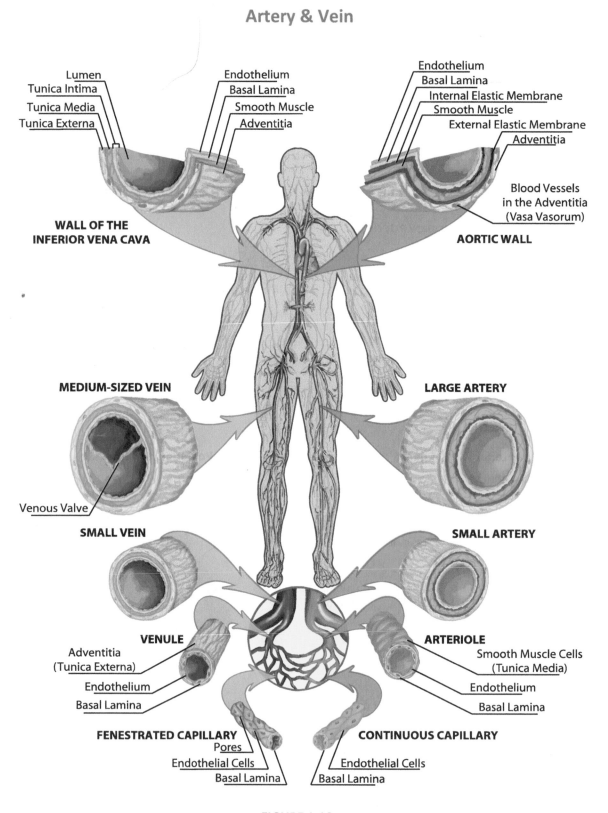

FIGURE 1.12

PROPERTIES OF CARDIAC TISSUE

Autorhythmicity: The ability to initiate a heart beat continuously and regularly without external stimulation. Rhythmicity is the ability of a tissue to produce its own impulses regularly. It is also called autorhythmicity or self-excitation.

Excitability: The ability to respond to a stimulus of adequate strength and duration (i.e. threshold or more) by generating a propagated action potential. Excitability is defined as the ability of a living tissue to give response to a stimulus.

Conductivity: The ability of cardiac cells to transfer the action potential generated at the sino-atrial node from cell to cell.

Contractility: The ability to contract in response to stimulation.

ANATOMICAL PLANES

Coronal Plane

Divides the body into front and back

Sagittal Plane

Divides the body into right and left

Horizontal or Transverse Plane

Divides the body into upper and lower parts

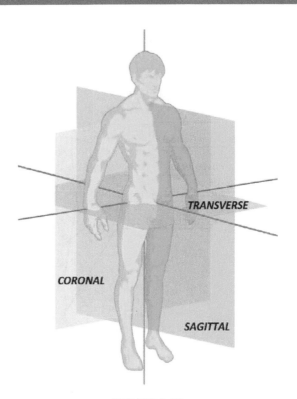

FIGURE 1.13

Chapter 1: ANATOMY & PHYSIOLOGY

Surface Anatomical Regions Front

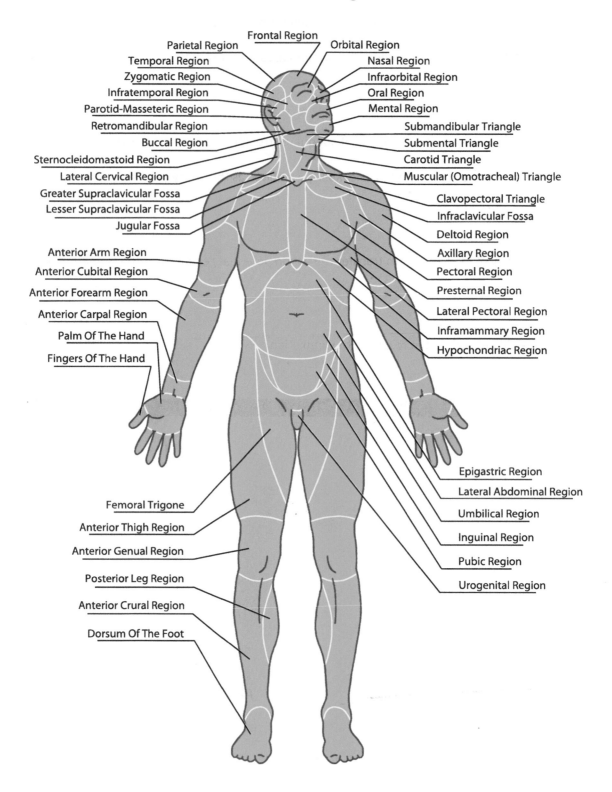

Parietal Region
Temporal Region
Zygomatic Region
Infratemporal Region
Parotid-Masseteric Region
Retromandibular Region
Buccal Region
Sternocleidomastoid Region
Lateral Cervical Region
Greater Supraclavicular Fossa
Lesser Supraclavicular Fossa
Jugular Fossa

Frontal Region
Orbital Region
Nasal Region
Infraorbital Region
Oral Region
Mental Region
Submandibular Triangle
Submental Triangle
Carotid Triangle
Muscular (Omotracheal) Triangle
Clavopectoral Triangle
Infraclavicular Fossa
Deltoid Region
Axillary Region
Pectoral Region
Presternal Region
Lateral Pectoral Region
Inframammary Region
Hypochondriac Region

Anterior Arm Region
Anterior Cubital Region
Anterior Forearm Region
Anterior Carpal Region
Palm Of The Hand
Fingers Of The Hand

Epigastric Region
Lateral Abdominal Region
Umbilical Region
Inguinal Region
Pubic Region
Urogenital Region

Femoral Trigone
Anterior Thigh Region
Anterior Genual Region
Posterior Leg Region
Anterior Crural Region
Dorsum Of The Foot

FIGURE 1.14

Chapter 1: ANATOMY & PHYSIOLOGY

Surface Anatomical Regions Back

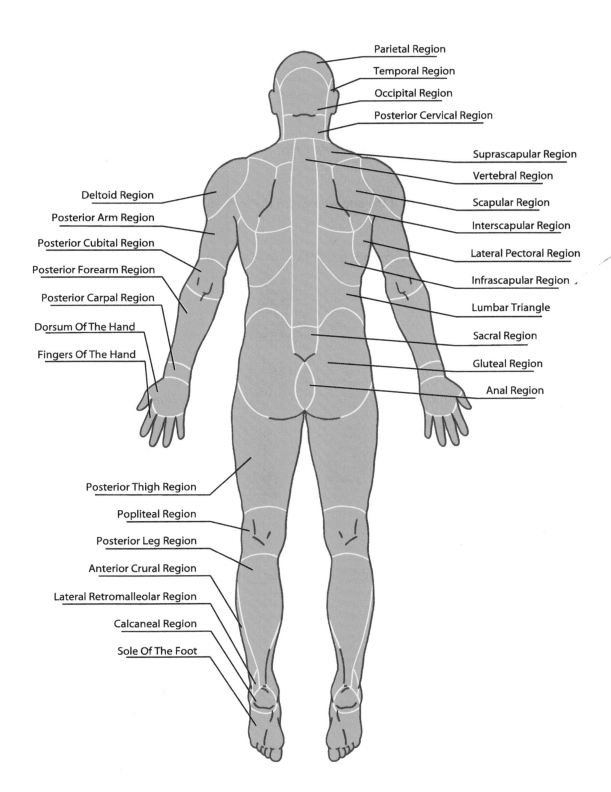

Parietal Region
Temporal Region
Occipital Region
Posterior Cervical Region
Suprascapular Region
Vertebral Region
Scapular Region
Interscapular Region
Lateral Pectoral Region
Infrascapular Region
Lumbar Triangle
Sacral Region
Gluteal Region
Anal Region

Deltoid Region
Posterior Arm Region
Posterior Cubital Region
Posterior Forearm Region
Posterior Carpal Region
Dorsum Of The Hand
Fingers Of The Hand
Posterior Thigh Region
Popliteal Region
Posterior Leg Region
Anterior Crural Region
Lateral Retromalleolar Region
Calcaneal Region
Sole Of The Foot

FIGURE 1.15

Medical Terminology

Medical terminology is language that is used to accurately describe the human body and associated

components, conditions and process.

ROOT:	most important as this is what gives the meaning to the whole term
SUFFIX:	this part is the one with which the term ends
PREFIX:	this part is the one with which the term starts
COMBINING VOWEL:	is what combines a root to another root, or a root to a suffix

Suffixes indicates	Prefix indicates
Procedure, Condition, Disorder, or Disease	Status, Time, Number and Location
Remember PCDD	**Remember STNL**

SUFFIX	PREFIX
Procedure : **graphy** (procedure that records)	Status : **dys** (means difficult, painful, or bad)
Condition : **algia** and **dynia** (pain)	Time : **pre** (before)
Disorder : **sclerosis** (abnormal hardening)	Number : **poly** (means many)
Disease : **pathy** (disease)	Location : **infra** (below or beneath)

Cardiovascular Terminology

Anastomosis

A surgical connection of two blood vessels.

Aneurysm

A localized thin & weakened area within a blood vessel.

Angiography

Procedure done to study the blood circulation of arteries.

Angioplasty

Is a procedure to widen a narrow or obstructed artery.

Aorta

Artery which carries oxygenated blood from the left ventricle to different parts of the body.

Aortic arch

The part of aorta that begins on the upper border of the aorta, from which arises arteries which carries blood to the upper parts of the body, and the downward curvature supplies blood to the rest of the body.

Aortic stenosis

Abnormal narrowing of the aortic valve.

Aortic valve

A valve present between the left ventricle and aorta, and prevents the back flow of blood from aorta back into the left ventricle.

Arrhythmia

Absence of rhythm in the heart beat.

Arterioles

Micro branches of arteries.

Artery

Carries oxygenated blood to different parts of the body starting from aorta.

Chapter 1: ANATOMY & PHYSIOLOGY

Arteriosclerosis

Thickening and hardening of the walls of the arteries.

Atrial fibrillation

Related to atria, unsynchronized contraction of atria.

Atrial flutter

Related to atria, abnormal beating, tachycardia (faster than usual).

Atrial septal defect (ASD)

Abnormal opening between the inter-atrial septum. *(between the right and left atrium)*

 ### Atrial septum

A wall present between the two upper chambers, dividing the atria into right and left atrium.

Atrioventricular block

Signals originating from atria that do not reach the ventricles.

Atrioventricular (AV) node

A pacemaker located at the boundaries of atria and ventricle and conducts impulse to the ventricle via the sino-atrial node.

 ### Brady

SLOW

 ### Bradycardia

SLOW HEART BEAT

Bundle-branch block

Defect is the electrical conduction system of the heart.

 ### Cardiac output

Amount of blood pumped by the heart in a minute.

Carotid artery

Artery that supplies blood to the brain via neck, this artery arises from the aorta.

Chapter 1: ANATOMY & PHYSIOLOGY

Co-arctation of the aorta

Narrowing of a part of the aorta.

 Conduction system

Pacemakers of the heart, SA node, AV node, Bundle of HIS, Purkinje Fibers.

Congenital

Existing at birth.

Congenital heart defect

A defect in the heart that is present at the time of birth.

Coronary arteries

Arteries that arises from the aorta and supplies the musculature of the heart.

Dextrocardia

 A condition in which the heart is on the right side of the chest.

 Diastole

Relaxation of the heart (ventricles) leading to filling of blood.

Ductus arteriosus

A condition in which a vessel connects the pulmonary artery to the aorta.

Dysrhythmia

Abnormal rhythm in the heart beat.

 Electrocardiogram (ECG or EKG)

A procedure done that records the electrical activity of the heart.

 Endocardium

The innermost layer of the heart.

Endocarditis

Inflammation with infection of the inner layer of the heart, usually with involvement of valves.

Chapter 1: ANATOMY & PHYSIOLOGY

Enlarged heart

Also called cardiomegaly, heart if bigger in size than normal.

Epicardium

 The outermost layer of the cardiac wall.

Exercise electrocardiogram (ECG or EKG)

A procedure done on a patient to record the electrical activity of the heart while the patient is performing an activity on a treadmill, bike or cycle ergometer.

Fibrillation

Unsynchronized contraction of heart muscles.

Flutter

Abnormal beating, tachycardia (faster than usual), synchronized contraction of heart muscles.

Heart block

Blockage of electrical impulse from one part to another within the heart.

 ### Holter monitor

A device attached to the patient for monitoring the activity of the heart for 24 to 48hours.

Hypoxemia

Reduced oxygen level in blood.

Hypoxia

Reduced oxygen level in tissues and cells of the body.

 ### Ischemia

Decrease in the blood flow to a part of the body due to obstruction in the artery carrying the blood to that region. Ischemia for long duration can lead to tissue death due to non-supply of oxygenated blood.

 ### Ischemic heart disease

Partial or Complete blockage of coronary arteries.

Chapter 1: ANATOMY & PHYSIOLOGY

Lumen

The passage present in the blood vessel through which the blood passes for maintaining circulation.

 Mitral valve

A type of atrio-ventricular valve present between the left atrium and left ventricle, prevents the back flow of blood from left ventricle back into left atrium. Also called as bicuspid valve.

 Myocardial infarction

Condition in which a part of the heart musculature is deprived of oxygenated blood for prolong time leading to death of the tissue.

 Myocardial ischemia

Decrease in the blood flow to a part of the body due to obstruction in the artery carrying the blood to that region. Ischemia for long duration can lead to tissue death due to non supply of oxygenated blood.

Myocarditis

Inflammation of mainly the myocardium.

 Myocardium

Middle layer of the heart which makes up the muscular portion of the atria and ventricles.

 Pacemaker (Artificial)

An artificial device which mimics an action of the natural pacemakers present in the heart.

Palpitation

Rapid beating or pounding of the heart.

Pericarditis

Inflammation of the pericardium.

 Pericardium

Thin double-layered sac which encloses and covers the heart.

Plaque

Build up of deposits causing partial or complete obstruction of blood flow within the artery.

Chapter 1: ANATOMY & PHYSIOLOGY

Pulmonary artery

An artery which carries the deoxygenated blood from the right ventricle into the right and left lung.

Pulmonary valve

A semilunar valve present between the right ventricle and the pulmonary artery.

Pulmonary vein

A vein which brings the oxygenated blood from the left and right lung into the left atrium.

 ### Septum

A muscular wall that divides the chambers of the heart.

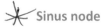 ### Sinus node

Natural pacemaker of the heart.

Sinus rhythm

Normal heart beat.

Sinus tachycardia

Faster heart beat which originates from sinus node.

 ### Sternum

The bone that is present in the midline of the thoracic cage anteriorly, it is divided into three parts: manubrium, body of sternum and xiphoid process.

Superior vena cava

A vein that returns the de-oxygenated blood from the body to the right atrium.

 ### Systole

The phase of the cardiac cycle in which the heart muscle contracts.

Systolic blood pressure

The pressure against the wall of the arteries during the contraction phase of the heart.

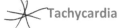 ### Tachycardia

Fast beating of the heart.

Chapter 1: ANATOMY & PHYSIOLOGY

Telemetry unit

A device which is used to monitor the EKG of a patient. In this the EKG signals are send in the form of waves from the transmitter unit to the receiver unit at a distant where it is being monitored for EKG.

Tetralogy of Fallot (TOF)

A complex congenital defect found at birth involving four heart defects.

Transposition of the great arteries

A congenital condition in which the aorta is connected to the right ventricle and pulmonary artery is connected to the left ventricle.

Tricuspid valve

An atrio-ventricular valve present between the right atrium and ventricle.

Valves

Are structures in heart which prevent the flow of blood in backward direction. Two type mainly atrioventricular and semilunar, which are further divided according to their locations.

Vasodilator

A prescription drug which causes dilation of the blood vessel due to relaxation of smooth muscles.

Vasopressor

A prescription drug which causes constriction of the blood vessel due to contraction of smooth muscles.

Vein

A blood vessel which carries deoxygenated blood. The only exception in the human body of a vein which carries oxygenated blood vessels is pulmonary vein.

Ventricle

Lower chambers of the heart, left and right ventricle.

Calculating Target Heart Rate & Maximum Heart Rate Using Karvonen Formula:

Step 1

220 - Age = Maximum Heart Rate

Step 2

Maximum Heart Rate(MHR) – Resting Heart Rate(RHR) = Heart Rate Reserve (HRR)

Step 3

Heart Rate Reserve (HRR) x Training Intensity % + Resting Heart Rate(RHR) = Training HR

Formula Summary

220 - _____ (your age) = _____ (your Max HR)

_____ (your Max HR) – _____ (your Resting HR) = _____ (HRR)

Use **HRR** below to get the desired heart rate.

Target Heart Rate Zone (50 to 65%) = Zone 1: Ranges from _____ to _____

50% = _____ (HRR) x 50% + _____ (rest HR) = _____ (50% training HR)
65% = _____ (HRR) x 65% + _____ (rest HR) = _____ (65% training HR)

Target Heart Rate Zone (60 to 75%) = Zone 2: Ranges from _____ to _____

60% = _____ (HRR) x 60% + _____ (rest HR) = _____ (60% training HR)
75% = _____ (HRR) x 75% + _____ (rest HR) = _____ (75% training HR)

Target Heart Rate Zone (70 to 85%) = Zone 3: Ranges from _____ to _____

70% = _____ (HRR) x 70% + _____ (rest HR) = _____ (70% training HR)
85% = _____ (HRR) x 85% + _____ (rest HR) = _____ (85% training HR)

Target Heart Rate Zone (80 to 95%) = Zone 4: Ranges from _____ to _____

80% = _____ (HRR) x 80% + _____ (rest HR) = _____ (80% training HR)
95% = _____ (HRR) x 95% + _____ (rest HR) = _____ (95% training HR)

Chapter 1: ANATOMY & PHYSIOLOGY

Example: A 40 year old woman with a resting heart rate (RHR) of 60bpm wants to train in Zone 3. Her HR training zones will be:

Karvonen Formula: 220 - 40 = 180 MHR

180 - 60 = 120 HRR

HR zones (70%): 120(0.70) + 60 = **144.0** (low end)

HR zones (85%): 120(0.85) + 60 = **162.0** (high end)

Calculate Zone 1, Zone 2, Zone 3, and Zone 4 for the following:

1. A 32 year old woman with a resting heart rate (RHR) of 67bpm
    Target Heart Rate Zone 1 (50 to 65%) = Zone 1: Ranges from _____ to _____
    Target Heart Rate Zone 2 (60 to 75%) = Zone 2: Ranges from _____ to _____
    Target Heart Rate Zone 3 (70 to 85%) = Zone 3: Ranges from _____ to _____
    Target Heart Rate Zone 4 (80 to 95%) = Zone 4: Ranges from _____ to _____

2. A 58 year old woman with a resting heart rate (RHR) of 70bpm
    Target Heart Rate Zone 1 (50 to 65%) = Zone 1: Ranges from _____ to _____
    Target Heart Rate Zone 2 (60 to 75%) = Zone 2: Ranges from _____ to _____
    Target Heart Rate Zone 3 (70 to 85%) = Zone 3: Ranges from _____ to _____
    Target Heart Rate Zone 4 (80 to 95%) = Zone 4: Ranges from _____ to _____

3. A 28 year old woman with a resting heart rate (RHR) of 69bpm
    Target Heart Rate Zone 1 (50 to 65%) = Zone 1: Ranges from _____ to _____
    Target Heart Rate Zone 2 (60 to 75%) = Zone 2: Ranges from _____ to _____
    Target Heart Rate Zone 3 (70 to 85%) = Zone 3: Ranges from _____ to _____
    Target Heart Rate Zone 4 (80 to 95%) = Zone 4: Ranges from _____ to _____

4. A 45 year old woman with a resting heart rate (RHR) of 65bpm
    Target Heart Rate Zone 1 (50 to 65%) = Zone 1: Ranges from _____ to _____
    Target Heart Rate Zone 2 (60 to 75%) = Zone 2: Ranges from _____ to _____
    Target Heart Rate Zone 3 (70 to 85%) = Zone 3: Ranges from _____ to _____
    Target Heart Rate Zone 4 (80 to 95%) = Zone 4: Ranges from _____ to _____

5. A 68 year old woman with a resting heart rate (RHR) of 73bpm
    Target Heart Rate Zone 1 (50 to 65%) = Zone 1: Ranges from _____ to _____
    Target Heart Rate Zone 2 (60 to 75%) = Zone 2: Ranges from _____ to _____
    Target Heart Rate Zone 3 (70 to 85%) = Zone 3: Ranges from _____ to _____
    Target Heart Rate Zone 4 (80 to 95%) = Zone 4: Ranges from _____ to _____

6. A 54 year old woman with a resting heart rate (RHR) of 74bpm
    Target Heart Rate Zone 1 (50 to 65%) = Zone 1: Ranges from _____ to _____
    Target Heart Rate Zone 2 (60 to 75%) = Zone 2: Ranges from _____ to _____
    Target Heart Rate Zone 3 (70 to 85%) = Zone 3: Ranges from _____ to _____
    Target Heart Rate Zone 4 (80 to 95%) = Zone 4: Ranges from _____ to _____

7. A 63 year old woman with a resting heart rate (RHR) of 63bpm
   Target Heart Rate Zone 1 (50 to 65%) = Zone 1: Ranges from _____ to _____
   Target Heart Rate Zone 2 (60 to 75%) = Zone 2: Ranges from _____ to _____
   Target Heart Rate Zone 3 (70 to 85%) = Zone 3: Ranges from _____ to _____
   Target Heart Rate Zone 4 (80 to 95%) = Zone 4: Ranges from _____ to _____

8. A 47 year old woman with a resting heart rate (RHR) of 75bpm
   Target Heart Rate Zone 1 (50 to 65%) = Zone 1: Ranges from _____ to _____
   Target Heart Rate Zone 2 (60 to 75%) = Zone 2: Ranges from _____ to _____
   Target Heart Rate Zone 3 (70 to 85%) = Zone 3: Ranges from _____ to _____
   Target Heart Rate Zone 4 (80 to 95%) = Zone 4: Ranges from _____ to _____

9. A 59 year old woman with a resting heart rate (RHR) of 77bpm
   Target Heart Rate Zone 1 (50 to 65%) = Zone 1: Ranges from _____ to _____
   Target Heart Rate Zone 2 (60 to 75%) = Zone 2: Ranges from _____ to _____
   Target Heart Rate Zone 3 (70 to 85%) = Zone 3: Ranges from _____ to _____
   Target Heart Rate Zone 4 (80 to 95%) = Zone 4: Ranges from _____ to _____

10. A 61 year old woman with a resting heart rate (RHR) of 68bpm
    Target Heart Rate Zone 1 (50 to 65%) = Zone 1: Ranges from _____ to _____
    Target Heart Rate Zone 2 (60 to 75%) = Zone 2: Ranges from _____ to _____
    Target Heart Rate Zone 3 (70 to 85%) = Zone 3: Ranges from _____ to _____
    Target Heart Rate Zone 4 (80 to 95%) = Zone 4: Ranges from _____ to _____

11. A 63 year old woman with a resting heart rate (RHR) of 65bpm
    Target Heart Rate Zone 1 (50 to 65%) = Zone 1: Ranges from _____ to _____
    Target Heart Rate Zone 2 (60 to 75%) = Zone 2: Ranges from _____ to _____
    Target Heart Rate Zone 3 (70 to 85%) = Zone 3: Ranges from _____ to _____
    Target Heart Rate Zone 4 (80 to 95%) = Zone 4: Ranges from _____ to _____

12. A 65 year old woman with a resting heart rate (RHR) of 66bpm
    Target Heart Rate Zone 1 (50 to 65%) = Zone 1: Ranges from _____ to _____
    Target Heart Rate Zone 2 (60 to 75%) = Zone 2: Ranges from _____ to _____
    Target Heart Rate Zone 3 (70 to 85%) = Zone 3: Ranges from _____ to _____
    Target Heart Rate Zone 4 (80 to 95%) = Zone 4: Ranges from _____ to _____

13. A 50 year old woman with a resting heart rate (RHR) of 69bpm
    Target Heart Rate Zone 1 (50 to 65%) = Zone 1: Ranges from _____ to _____
    Target Heart Rate Zone 2 (60 to 75%) = Zone 2: Ranges from _____ to _____
    Target Heart Rate Zone 3 (70 to 85%) = Zone 3: Ranges from _____ to _____
    Target Heart Rate Zone 4 (80 to 95%) = Zone 4: Ranges from _____ to _____

14. A 49 year old woman with a resting heart rate (RHR) of 70bpm
    Target Heart Rate Zone 1 (50 to 65%) = Zone 1: Ranges from _____ to _____
    Target Heart Rate Zone 2 (60 to 75%) = Zone 2: Ranges from _____ to _____
    Target Heart Rate Zone 3 (70 to 85%) = Zone 3: Ranges from _____ to _____
    Target Heart Rate Zone 4 (80 to 95%) = Zone 4: Ranges from _____ to _____

Chapter 1: ANATOMY & PHYSIOLOGY

End of Chapter Review

1. The Heart is a muscular organ that is situated in the ___Mediastinum___

2. Which of the following are not the boundaries of the mediastinum?

    a) ___Superiorly (thoracic inlet)

    b) ___Inferiorly (diaphragm)

    c) ✓Medially (bodies of thoracic vertebrae)

    d) ___Laterally (mediastinal pleura)

3. The Heart is made up of four chambers, __two Atria__ and__two ventricles__

4. _Force of Contraction_ of the heart depends on the muscle size.

5. Right side of the heart has two chambers, _Right Atrium_ and _Right ventricle_

6. The Right atrium consists of the pacemaker known as _Sino-Atrial Node_ that produces cardiac impulses

    and _Atrio-ventricular_ Node which is present at the boundaries between the _Atria_ and ____

    ventricles that conducts the impulses to the _ventricles_.

7. The Right atrium receives __DEOXYgenated__ (venous) blood

8. _Superior vena cava_ that returns venous blood from the head, neck and upper limbs

9. Inferior vena cava that returns __venous__ from lower parts of the body

10. The Right atrium communicates with the right ventricle through the _tricuspid_ valve.

11. From the right ventricle, __pulmonary__ artery arises.

12. In the lungs, the __deoxygenated__ blood is oxygenated.

13. The Left side of the heart has two chambers, the __Left atrium__ and the _Left ventricle_

14. The left atrium receives oxygenated blood from the lungs through _Pulmonary veins_

15. Blood from left atrium enters the left ventricle through the__bicuspid__ valve.

16. The right atrioventricular valve is known as the _tricuspid_ valve.

Chapter 1: ANATOMY & PHYSIOLOGY

17. The left atrioventricular valve is called __Mitral__ valve.

18. Cusps of the valves are attached to __papillary muscles__ by means of the chordate tendineae.

19. __papillary Muscles__ play an important role in the closure of the cusps and in preventing the back flow of blood from the ventricle to the atria during ventricular contraction.

20. __Atrioventricular__ valves open only towards the ventricles and prevent the backflow of blood into the atria.

21. The right and left atria are separated from one another by a fibrous septum called __inter Atrial septum__

22. The right and left ventricles are separated from one another by __inter-Ventricular septum__

23. Which of the following is not a layer of the heart?

    a) ___Pericardium

    b) ___Myocardium

    c) ___Endocardium

    d) √ Intercardium

24. __Systemic Ciculation__ is otherwise known as greater circulation.

25. __Pulmonary Ciculation__ is otherwise called lesser circulation.

26. During ventricular diastole, heart relaxes and blood from the right atrium is filled into the __Right Ventricle__ by opening of __Tricuspid__ valve and blood from the __Left Atrium__ is filled into the left ventricle by opening of the __Mitral__ _or bicuspid_ valve.

27. During ventricular systole, ventricles contracts and pumps the blood from the __Right Ventricle__ into the pulmonary artery with closure of the __tricuspid__ valve and opening of the __pulmonary valve__ and from the left ventricle into the __Aorta__ with closure of the __bicuspid or Mitral__ valve and opening of aortic valve.

28. __Stroke Volume__ is the amount of blood pumped out by each ventricle during each beat.

29. _Heart Rate_ is the number of times the heart beats in one minute.

30. _Cardiac Output_ is the amount of blood pumped out by each ventricle in one minute.

31. Cardiac Output (CO) = _Stroke Volume_ × _Heart Rate_

32. A person with heart rate of 72 and stroke volume of 70 will have a cardiac output of _5040_ ml/min

33. All of the following are pacemakers of the heart except

    a) ___ Sino-Atrial Node (SA Node)

    b) ___ Atrio-Ventricular Node (AV Node)

    c) ___ Bundle of His

    d) _✓_ Sinus Rhythm

34. Heart muscle is supplied by two coronary arteries, namely _Right_ and _Left Coronary_ arteries, which are the first branches of aorta.

35. Right coronary artery supplies whole of the _Right_ ventricle and posterior portion of left _ventricle_

36. Left coronary artery supplies mainly the _Anterior_ and lateral parts of left _ventricle_.

37. _Autorhythmicity_ is the ability to initiate a heart beat continuously and regularly without external stimulation.

38. _Excitability_ is the ability to respond to a stimulus of adequate strength and duration

39. _Conductivity_ is the ability of cardiac cells to transfer the action potential generated at the sino-atrial node from cell to cell.

40. _Contractility_ is the ability to contract in response to stimulation.

41. Sagittal Plane divides the body into _Right_ and _Left_

42. Coronal Plane divides the body into _Front_ and _back_

43. Horizontal or Transverse Plane divides the body into _upper_ and _Lower_

Chapter 1: ANATOMY & PHYSIOLOGY

44. _Angioplasty_ is a procedure to widen a narrow or obstructed artery.

45. _Aorta_ is an artery which carries oxygenated blood from the left ventricle to different parts of the body.

46. _Aortic Stenosis_ means abnormal narrowing of the aortic valve.

47. _Artery_ carries oxygenated blood to different parts of the body starting from aorta.

48. _Arteriosclerosis_ is the thickening and hardening of the walls of the arteries.

49. _Atrial septal defect_ is an abnormal opening between the interatrial septum. (between the right and left atrium)

50. _Atrial Septum_ is a wall present between the two upper chambers, dividing the atria into right and left atrium.

51. _Dextrocardia_ is a condition in which the heart is on the right side of the chest.

52. _Enlarged heart_ is also called cardiomegaly, heart if bigger in size than normal.

53. _Hypoxemia_ is due to reduced oxygen level in blood.

54. _Hypoxia_ is due to reduced oxygen level in tissues and cells of the body.

55. _Ischemia_ is due to decrease in the blood flow to a part of the body due to obstruction in the artery carrying the blood to that region. Ischemia for long duration can lead to tissue death due to non supply of oxygenated blood.

56. _Myocardial Infarction_ is a condition in which a part of the heart musculature is deprived of oxygenated blood for prolong time leading to death of the tissue.

57. _Ischemia_ is a decrease in the blood flow to a part of the body due to obstruction in the artery carrying the blood to that region

58. A _Semi Lunar_ valve is present between the right ventricle and the pulmonary artery.

59. _Vein_ is a blood vessel which carries deoxygenated blood.

Chapter 1: ANATOMY & PHYSIOLOGY

60. LABLE THE DIAGRAM 1.1

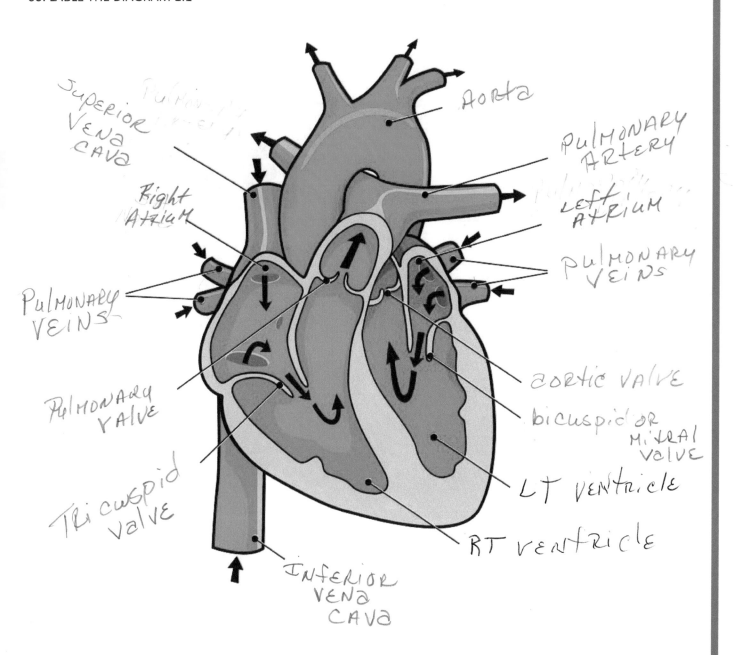

CHAPTER 2

ELECTROCARDIOGRAPHY THEORY

Electrocardiography

Electrocardiography is a **procedure** by which the electrical activities of the heart are recorded. The spread

of excitation throughout the myocardium cells produce electrical potential, this potential causes a current

flow, which acts as a **volume conductor.** This current produced can be picked up from the surface of the

body by using electrodes which receives and sends the recording to the electrocardiogram for recording in

the form of waves. The procedure was discovered by, **Willem Einthoven.**

Electrocardiograph

Electrocardiograph is the **instrument** (machine) by which electrical activities of the heart are recorded.

Electrocardiogram

Electrocardiogram (EKG or ECG) is the **graphical representation** of electrical activities of the heart.

USES OF EKG

Electrocardiogram is useful in determining and diagnosing the following:

1. Heart rate

2. Heart rhythm

3. Heart attack

4. Poor blood flow to heart muscle (ischemia)

5. Abnormal electrical conduction

6. Coronary artery disease

7. Hypertrophy of heart chambers or axis deviation of heart

EKG LEADS

EKG leads record graphical representation of waves PQRST on a graph paper. These leads are called

EKG leads and are generated by the EKG machine. Heart is said to be in the center of an **equilateral**

triangle drawn by connecting the roots of these three limbs. This creates a triangle called **Einthoven**

Triangle. (Refer Figure 2.1)

Einthoven Triangle and Einthoven Law

Einthoven triangle is defined as an equilateral triangle that is used as a model of standard limb leads used

to record electrocardiogram. Heart is presumed to lie in the center of einthovens triangle. Electrical

potential generated from the heart appears simultaneously on the roots of the three limbs, namely the

left arm, right arm and the left leg.

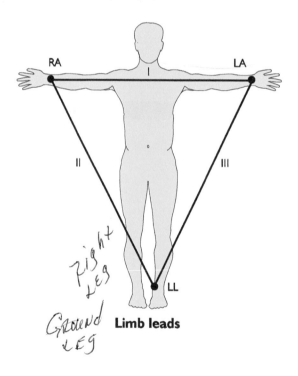

FIGURE 2.1

Chapter 2: EKG THEORY

EKG is recorded in 12 leads, which are generally classified into two categories.

I. Bipolar leads

II. Unipolar leads

BIPOLAR LIMB LEADS

Bipolar limb leads are otherwise known as **standard limb leads (SLL).**

Standard limb leads are:

a. *Limb Lead I*

b. *Limb Lead II*

c. *Limb Lead III*

[handwritten: RT ARM − , LT ARM +, RT ARM − , LT Leg +, LT ARM − , LT Leg +]

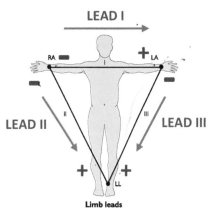

FIGURE 2.1a

Lead I

Lead I is generated by connecting right arm and left arm.

Right arm is connected to the negative terminal and the left arm is connected to the

positive terminal.

Lead II

Lead II is generated by connecting right arm and left leg. Right arm is connected to the negative terminal

and the left leg is connected to the positive terminal.

Lead III

Lead III is generated by connecting left arm and left leg. Left arm is connected to the negative terminal

and the left leg is connected to the positive terminal.

BIPOLAR LIMB LEADS

Standard Limb Leads are of three types:

a. **Limb Lead I** = **LA (POSITIVE ELECTRODE)** + RA (NEGATIVE ELECTRODE)

b. **Limb Lead II** = **LL (POSITIVE ELECTRODE)** + RA (NEGATIVE ELECTRODE)

c. **Limb Lead III** = **LL (POSITIVE ELECTRODE)** + LA (NEGATIVE ELECTRODE)

UNIPOLAR LEADS

In unipolar leads one electrode in an **active electrode** and the other is an **indifferent electrode.**

Unipolar leads are:

1. Unipolar limb leads (ULL)

2. Unipolar chest leads (UCL)

1. Unipolar Limb Leads

Unipolar limb leads are also called **Augmented Unipolar Limb Leads.**

Augmented Unipolar Limb Leads are:

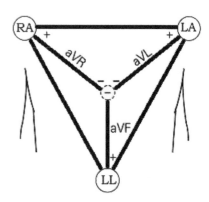

1. aVR lead : Active electrode is directed towards the right arm

2. aVL lead : Active electrode is directed towards the left arm

3. aVF lead : Active electrode is directed towards the left leg (foot)

FIGURE 2.2

2. *Unipolar Chest Leads*

Chest leads are denoted as **'V' leads** or **precordial chest leads.**

Active electrode is placed on six different locations over the chest. These electrodes are known as the chest electrodes and the six locations over the chest are called **V1, V2, V3, V4, V5** and **V6**.

"**V**" indicates vector, which shows the direction of current flow.

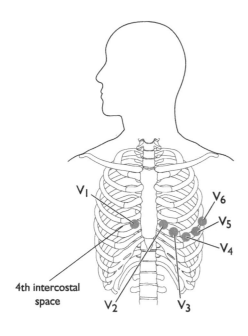 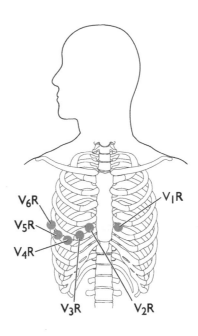

A. Standard chest lead placement   **B. Right sided chest lead placement**

FIGURE 2.3

Position of chest leads:

V1 : Over 4th intercostal space near right sternal margin

V2 : Over 4th intercostal space near left sternal margin

V3 : In between V2 and V4

V4 : Over left 5th intercostal space on the left mid clavicular line

V5 : Over left 5th intercostal space on the left anterior axillary line

V6 : Over left 5th intercostal space on the left mid axillary line.

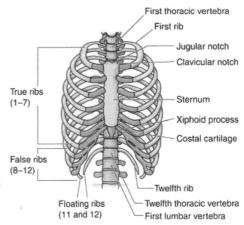

FIGURE 2.4

ECG and electrical activity of the myocardium

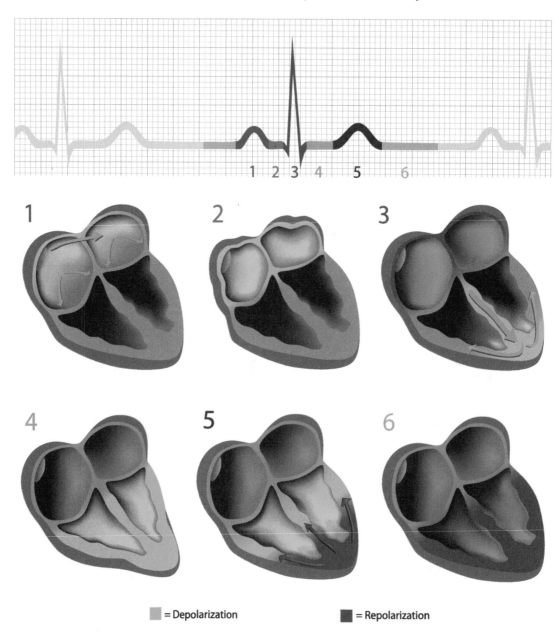

= Depolarization   = Repolarization

FIGURE 2.5

12 LEAD EKG (ELECTRODES)

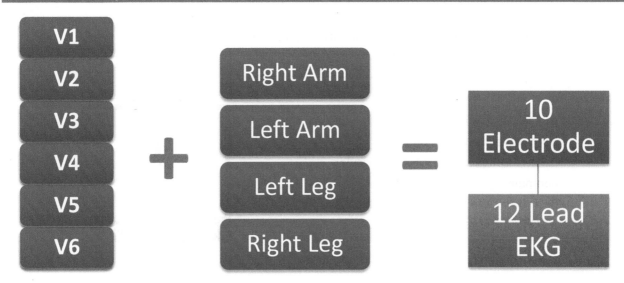

12 LEAD EKG (LEAD POLARITY)

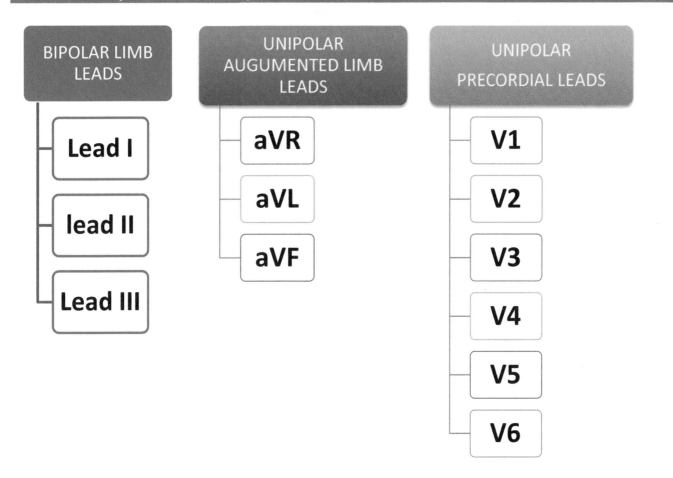

WAVES OF NORMAL EKG

Normal EKG consists of waves, complexes, intervals and segments.

Normal electrocardiogram has the following waves, namely P, Q, R, S and T.

The letter **PQRST** was chosen by Einthoven instead of regular alphabets ABCDE.

Major Complexes in ECG
1. 'P' wave, the atrial complex
2. 'QRS' complex, the initial ventricular complex
3. 'T' wave, the final ventricular complex
4. 'QRST', the ventricular complex.

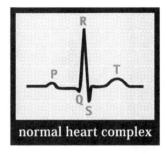

normal heart complex

FIGURE 2.6

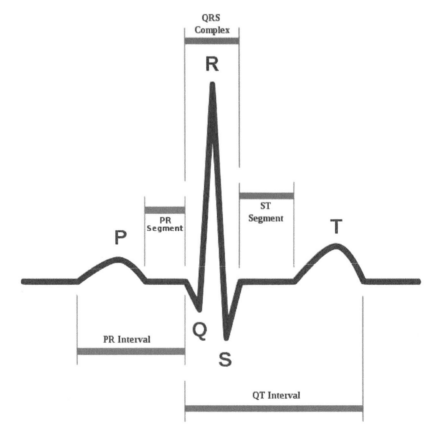

FIGURE 2.7

ELECTROCARDIOGRAPHIC GRID

The paper that is used for recording EKG is called EKG paper. EKG machine amplifies the electrical signals produced from the heart and records these signals on a moving EKG paper. Electrocardiographic grid refers to the graphs on the EKG paper. EKG paper has horizontal lines and vertical lines at regular intervals of 1 millimeter (mm).

DURATION

Time duration of EKG waves is plotted horizontally on X-axis.

On X-axis

Small Box = 0.04 second

Large Box = 0.20 second

AMPLITUDE

Amplitude of EKG waves is plotted vertically on Y-axis.

On Y-axis

Small Box = 0.1 mV

Large Box = 0.5 mV

SPEED OF THE PAPER

Movement of paper through the machine can be adjusted by two speeds, 25 mm/second and 50 mm/second. Usually, speed of the paper during recording is fixed at 25 mm/second. If heart rate is very high, speed of the paper is changed to 50 mm/second.*(for e.g tachycardia or pediatrics)*

DURATION X-AXIS	AMPLITUDE: Y-AXIS	SPEED
• Small Box 0.04 second • Large Box 0.20 second	• Small Box 1mm = 0.1mv • Large Box 5mm = 0.5mv	• 25mm/second • 50mm/second

TABLE 2.1

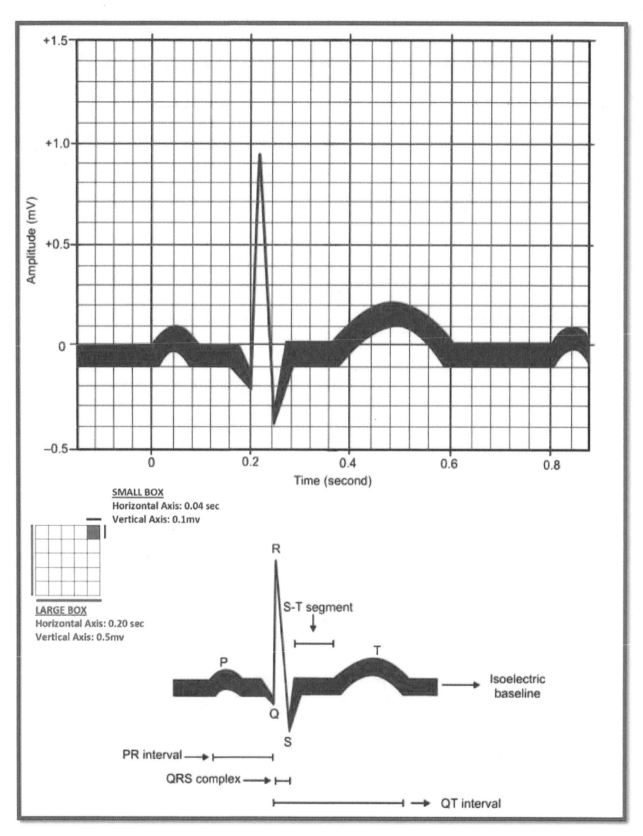

SMALL BOX
Horizontal Axis: 0.04 sec
Vertical Axis: 0.1mv

LARGE BOX
Horizontal Axis: 0.20 sec
Vertical Axis: 0.5mv

FIGURE 2.8

Chapter 2: EKG THEORY

P WAVE

'P' wave is a first positive wave seen in the EKG.

It is also called **atrial complex wave.**

Cause

'P' wave is produced due to the **depolarization**

of **atria of the heart (upper two chambers).**

Depolarization spreads from Sino-Atrial node to

all parts of atria. **Atrial repolarization** is not

recorded as a separate wave in EKG because it

takes place at the same time as that of the ventricular

activity (QRS complex).

Morphology

'P' wave is normally positive & upright in leads I,

II, aVF, V4, V5 and V6.

It is normally negative (inverted) in aVR. It is

variable in the remaining leads, i.e. it may be

positive, negative, biphasic or flat

Clinical Significance

Variation in the duration, amplitude and

morphology of 'P' wave helps in the diagnosis of

several cardiac problems such as:

1. *Right atrial hypertrophy*

2. *Left atrial dilatation or hypertrophy*

3. *Atrial extrasystole*

4. *Hyperkalemia*

5. *Atrial fibrillation*

6. *Middle AV nodal rhythm*

7. *Sinoatrial block*

8. *Atrial paroxysmal tachycardia*

9. *Lower AV nodal rhythm*

QRS COMPLEX

'QRS' complex is the **ventricular complex.**

"Q" wave is a negative wave

"R" wave is the next wave which is positive

"S" wave is the next negative wave after "R"

Cause

'QRS' complex is due to **depolarization** of

ventricular chambers of the heart.

'Q' wave is due to the depolarization **(basal**

portion) of interventricular septum .

'R' wave is due to the depolarization **(apical**

portion) of interventricular septum and the

ventricular musculature.

'S' wave is represents the final depolarization of

basal portion of ventricular musculature.

Duration

Normal duration of 'QRS' complex is between

0.06 and 0.10 second.(*may vary*)

Morphology

'Q' wave is usually small with amplitude of 4 mm

or less. It is less than 25 percent of amplitude of

'R' waves in leads I, II, aVL, V5 and V6.

 From chest leads V1 to V6, 'R' wave becomes

gradually larger. It is smaller in V6 than V5.

'S' wave is large in V1 and larger in V2. It

gradually becomes smaller from V3 to V6.

Clinical Significance

Variation in the duration, amplitude and

morphology of 'QRS' complex helps in the

diagnosis of several cardiac problems such as:

1. *Bundle branch block*

2. *Hyperkalemia*

T WAVE

'T' wave is a positive wave.

Cause

'T' wave is due to the **repolarization (relaxation)** of **ventricular muscles.**

Morphology

 'T' wave is normally positive in leads I, II, V5 and V6.

It is normally inverted in lead aVR.

Clinical Significance

Variation in duration, amplitude and morphology of 'T' wave helps in the diagnosis of several cardiac problems such as:

1. Acute myocardial ischemia

2. Age

3. Myocardial infarction

4. Left ventricular hypertrophy

3. Hypokalemia

4. Hyperkalemia

U WAVE

 'U' wave is not always seen. It is also an insignificant wave in EKG. It is supposed to be due to **repolarization** of **papillary muscle or Purkinje fibers.**

Clinical Significance

Appearance of 'U' wave in EKG indicates some clinical conditions such as:

1. *Hypercalcemia, thyrotoxicosis and hypokalemia:* 'U' wave appears. It is very prominent in hypokalemia.

2. *Myocardial ischemia:* Inverted 'U' wave appears.

P-R INTERVAL

'**P-R**' interval is the interval from the start of '**P**' wave to the start of '**Q**' wave.

'**P-R**' interval signifies the conduction of impulses through AV node. It shows the duration of conduction of the impulses from the SA node to ventricles through atrial musculature and AV node.

'**P**' wave represents the atrial depolarization. Short period on the iso-electric line after the end of '**P**' wave represents the time taken for the passage of depolarization to the AV node.

Duration

Normal duration of '**P-R interval**' is 0.18 second and varies between 0.12 and 0.20 second. If it is more than 0.20 second, it signifies the delay in the conduction of impulse from SA node to the ventricles.

Clinical Significance

Variation in the duration of '**P-R**' intervals helps in the diagnosis of several cardiac problems such as:

1. Bradycardia

2. First degree heart block

3. Tachycardia

Q-T INTERVAL

'**Q-T**' interval is the interval from the start of the '**Q**' wave to the end of '**T**' wave.

'**Q-T**' interval indicates the ventricular depolarization and ventricular repolarization. It shows the electrical activity taking place in the ventricles.

Clinical Significance

Prolong Q-T
1. Myocardial infarction
2. Myocarditis
3. Hypocalcemia
4. Hypothyroidism

Shorten Q-T
1. Hypercalcemia

S-T SEGMENT

'**S-T**' segment is the interval between the end of the '**S**' wave to the onset of '**T**' wave. ST segment is the isoelectric period.

Duration of 'S-T' Segment

Normal duration of '**S-T**' segment is around 0.08 second.

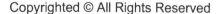

Clinical Significance Variation in the duration of '**S-T**' segment and its deviation from isoelectric line indicates the pathological conditions such as:
1. Myocardial infarction
2. Left bundle branch block
3. Pericarditis
4. Athletes
5. Myocardial ischemia
6. Ventricular hypertrophy
7. Hypokalemia
8. Hypocalcemia
9. Hypercalcemia

A – Dε-C   Rε – Rε   V· Dε-C

UNDERSTANDING THE WAVES

What is a P Waves	Atrial Depolarization	Contraction
What is a Q Waves	Ventricular Depolarization	Contraction
What is a R Waves	Ventricular Depolarization	Contraction
What is a S Waves	Ventricular Depolarization	Contraction
What is a T Waves	Ventricular Repolarization	Relaxation

TABLE 2.2

MEASURING THE COMPLEX , INTERVAL & SEGMENT

QRS Complex	Start of Q waves to the End of S wave
PR Interval	Start of P waves to the Start of Q wave
QT Interval	Start of Q waves to the End of T wave
ST Segment	End of S waves to the Start of T wave

TABLE 2.3

CRITERIAS FOR GRAPH INTERPRETATION

QRS	Normal, Wide or Narrow
PR	Normal, Prolong or Shortened
QT	Normal, Prolong or Shortened
ST	Normal, Elevation or Depression
P Waves before every QRS COMPLEX	Present or Absent

TABLE 2.4

CALCULATING HEART RATE

REGULAR GRAPH	IRREGULAR GRAPH
300 METHOD (Approximate) 300/Number of Large Box Between 2 R waves	**6 Second Method** 30 Large Boxes X 0.20 Sec = 6 Sec Calculate number of R waves X 10 = __ HR
1500 METHOD (Accurate) 1500/Number of Small Box Between 2 R waves	

TABLE 2.5

POINTS TO LOOK FOR IN A EKG TEST STRIP (WAVES)

		If Present		If Absent	Result
P Wave	Is the P wave Present?	If Present What is the Duration: MM:? MV:?	1. Is it Normal 2. Normal 2.5mm & 0.12sec *may vary*	If Absent No Atrial Depolarization Took Place	Result _____
Q Wave	Is the Q wave Present?	If Present What is the Duration: MM:? MV:?	Is it Normal	If Absent Ventricular Septum Depolarization Absent	Result _____
R Wave	Is the R wave Present?	If Present What is the Duration: MM:? MV:?	Is it Normal	If Absent No Ventricular Depolarization Took Place	Result _____
S Wave	Is the S wave Present?	If Present What is the Duration: MM:? MV:?	Is it Normal	If Absent No Ventricular Depolarization Took Place (Basal Portion)	Result _____
T Wave	Is the T wave Present?	If Present What is the Duration: MM:? MV:?	Is it Normal	If Absent No Ventricular Repolarization Took Place (Purkinje Fibers)	Result _____

TABLE 2.6

Notes:_____

_____

_____

_____

_____

_____

_____

_____

_____

POINTS TO LOOK FOR IN A EKG TEST STRIP (COMPLEX)

STEP 1	STEP 2	STEP 3	STEP 4	
QRS Complex	Is the QRS Complex Present? If Yes What is the Duration:? *Normal Duration 0.06sec - 0.10sec* *may vary*	Is the QRS Complex in Normal Ranges of duration If Yes 1. Check for Individual Waves 2. Identify Individual Waves Q: Present or Absent R: Present or Absent S: Present or Absent	If Narrow QRS Complex : Less than Normal duration If Wider QRS Complex: More than Normal duration	Result

TABLE 2.7

Notes:_____

_____

_____

_____

_____

_____

_____

_____

_____

_____

_____

_____

_____

_____

_____

_____

_____

_____

POINTS TO LOOK FOR IN A EKG TEST STRIP (SEGMENT)

STEP 1	STEP 2	STEP 3	STEP 4	
ST Segment	Is the ST Segment Present? If Yes • Is it Normal • Is it Elevated • Is it Depressed	Is the ST Segment in Normal Ranges of duration *Normal Duration 0.08sec (2 small boxes)* *may vary*	If Narrow ST Segment : Less than Normal duration If Wider ST Segment : More than Normal duration	Result

TABLE 2.8

POINTS TO LOOK FOR IN A EKG TEST STRIP (INTERVAL)

STEP 1	STEP 2	STEP 3	STEP 4	
PR Interval	Is the PR Interval Present? If Yes What is the Duration:	Is the PR Interval in Normal Ranges of duration *Normal Duration 0.12sec - 0.20sec (3-5 small boxes)* *may vary*	If Narrow PR Interval : Less than Normal duration If Wider PR Interval : More than Normal duration	Result
QT Interval	Is the QT Interval Present? If Yes What is the Duration:	Is the QT Interval in Normal Ranges of duration *Normal Duration 0.40sec (2 large boxes)* *may vary*	If Narrow QT Interval : Less than Normal duration If Wider QT Interval : More than Normal duration	Result

TABLE 2.9

Notes:_____

_____

_____

R-R INTERVAL

'**R-R**' interval is the time interval between two consecutive '**R**' waves.

Significance

'**R-R**' interval signifies the duration of one cardiac cycle.

Significance of Measuring 'R-R' Interval

Measurement of '**R-R**' interval helps to calculate:

Heart Rate

Calculation of heart rate

Two types of EKG Rhythms:

1. Regular Rhythm Graph

To get an approximate heart rate, count the number of larger boxes between R-R waves

- **Use the formula:** 300 ÷ number of large boxes on the EKG graph paper between 2 R waves = **Heart Rate**
  For e.g number of large boxes between R-R waves is 3, **300 ÷ 3 = 100 Heart Rate**

To get an accurate heart rate, count the number of small boxes between R-R waves

- **Use the formula:** 1500 ÷ number of small boxes on the EKG graph paper between 2 R waves = **Heart Rate**
  For e.g number of small boxes between R-R waves is 12, **1500 ÷ 12 = 125 Heart Rate**

2. Irregular Rhythm Graph

Count the number of R waves in 30 large boxes (6 second rhythm strip)

- Multiply the number of R waves in a 6 second rhythm strip by **10** to get the **Heart Rate**
  For e.g **R waves** in a 6 second rhythm strip are **8**, by using the formula
  Calculation: 8 (number of R waves in a 6 second rhythm strip) × **10 = 80** Heart Rate

EKG GRAPH INTERPRETATION

Rhythm Originating from Sinus Node

1. Normal Sinus Rhythm

2. Sinus Bradycardia

3. Sinus Tachycardia

4. Sinus Arrhythmia

5. Sinus Pause/Sinus Arrest

Rhythms Originating from the Atrial-Junction Node

1. Junctional Rhythm

2. Supraventricular Tachycardia

Heart Blocks

1. First Degree

2. Second Degree Type 1

3. Second Degree Type 2

4. Third Degree

Rhythm Originating from Atria's

1. Sino-Atrial Block

2. Premature Atrial Complex

3. Wandering Atrial Pacemaker

4. Atrial Flutter

5. Atrial Fibrillation

Rhythms Originating from the Ventricles

1. Idioventricular Rhythm

2. Ventricular Fibrillation

3. Premature Ventricular Contraction

4. Torsades de pointes

5. Asystole

6. Ventricular Tachycardia

EKG analysis consists of a five-step process of gathering data about each rhythm strip. These steps include evaluating the following components of the EKG rhythm strips:

- Rhythm (regularity)

- Rate

- QRS duration and configuration

- P wave configuration

- PR interval

Normal Sinus Rhythm

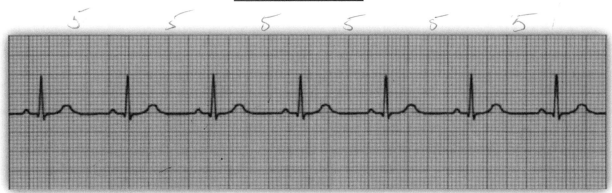

Figure 2.9

Sinus Bradycardia

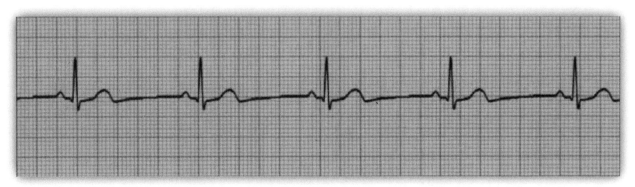

Figure 2.10

Sinus Tachycardia

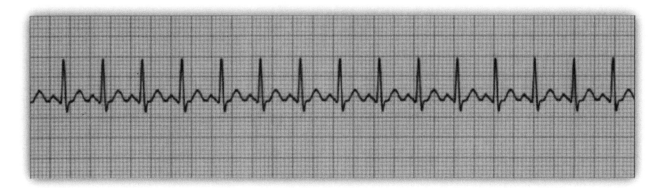

Figure 2.11

Rhythm chANge

Sinus Arrhythmia

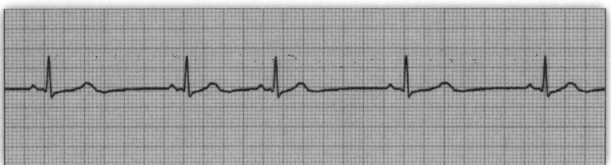

Figure 2.12

Big Bridge

Sinus Pause

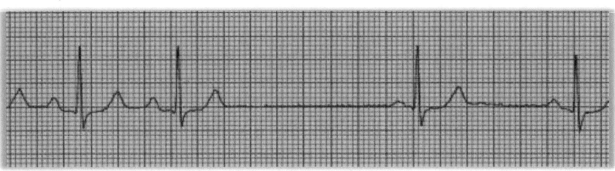

Figure 2.13

SmAll Bridge

Sino-Atrial Block

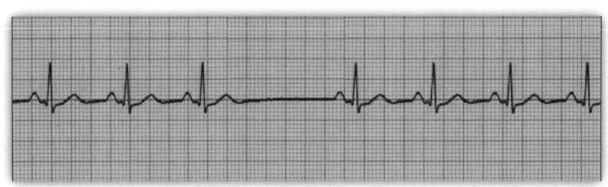

Figure 2.14

Premature Atrial Contraction

lit w
pig w

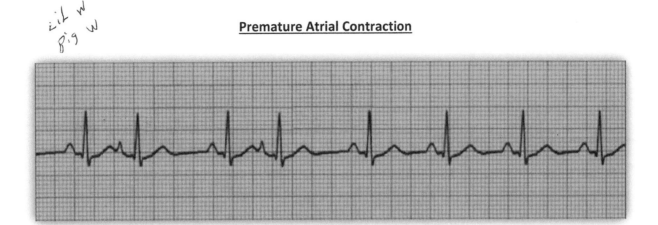

Figure 2.15

Wandering Atrial Pacemaker

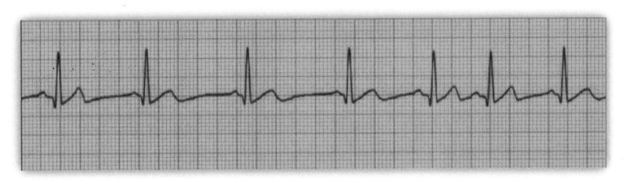

Figure 2.16

Atrial Flutter

shark Teeth   *WATER*

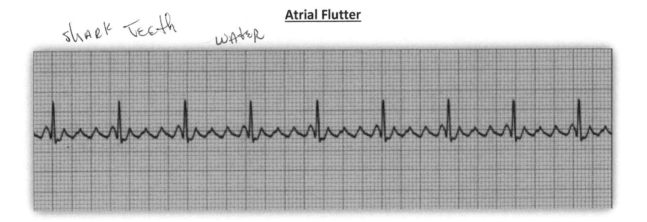

Figure 2.17

Atrial Fibrillation

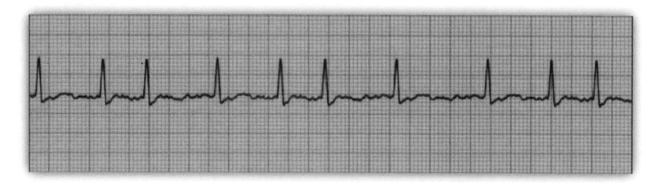

Figure 2.18

Junctional Rhythm (Escape)

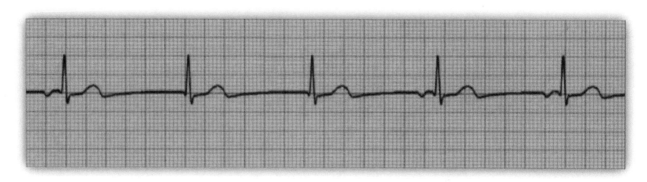

Figure 2.19

Supraventricular Tachycardia

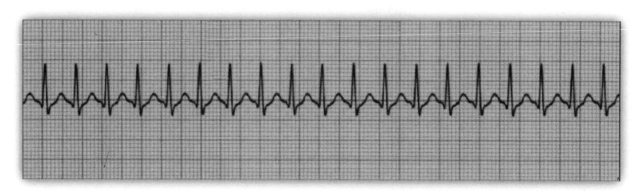

Figure 2.20

First Degree Block

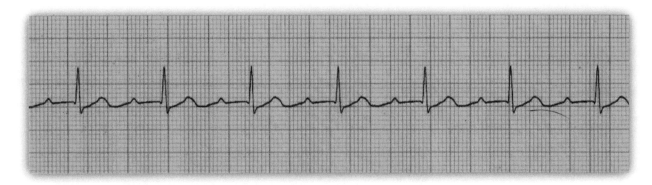

Figure 2.21

Second Degree Block Type 1: Mobitz I or Wenckebach

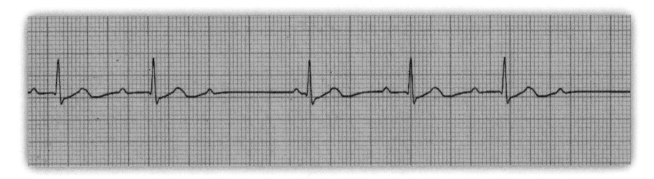

Figure 2.22

Second Degree Block Type 2 (Mobitz II)

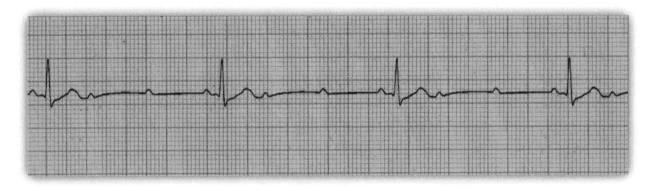

Figure 2.23

Third Degree Block (Complete Heart Block)

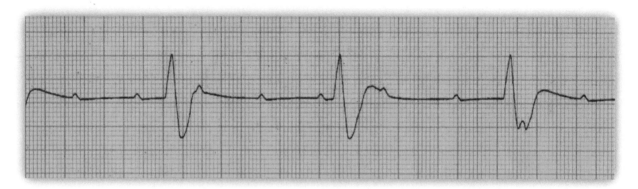

Figure 2.24

Idioventricular Rhythm

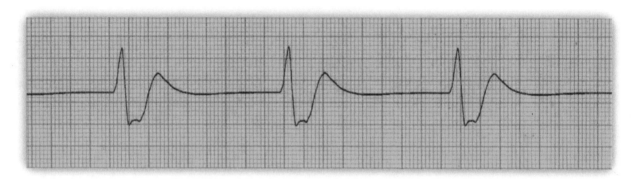

Figure 2.25

Ventricular Fibrillation

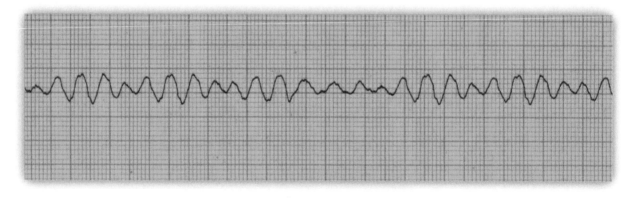

Figure 2.26

Premature Ventricular Contraction

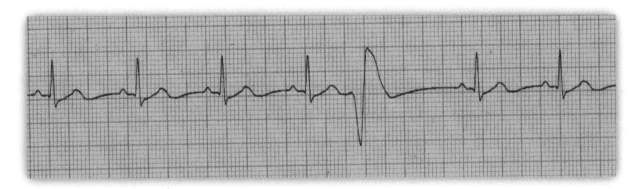

Figure 2.27

Asystole

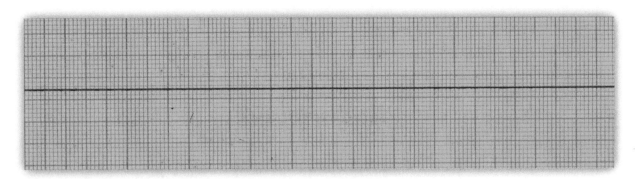

Figure 2.28

Ventricular Tachycardia

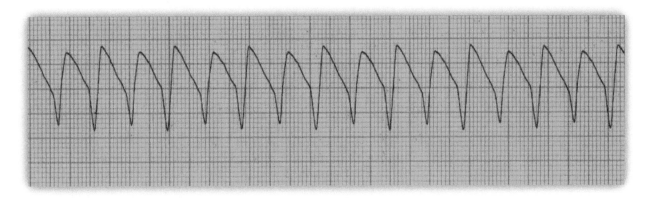

Figure 2.29

Torsades de pointes

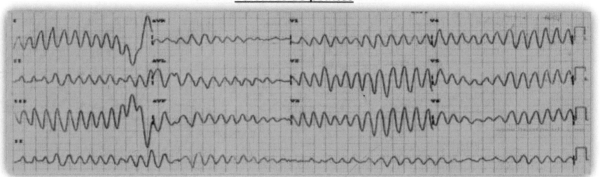

Figure 2.30

MUSCLE ARTIFACTS

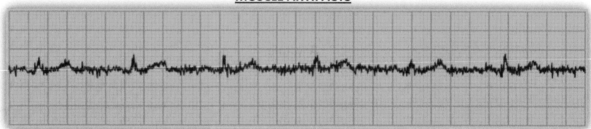

Figure 2.31

60 CYCLE INTERFERENCE

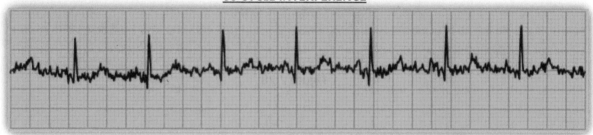

Figure 2.32

RESPIRATION

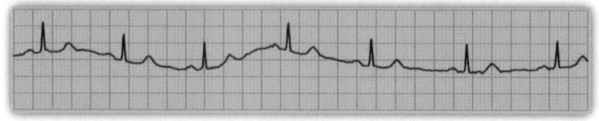

Figure 2.33

Chapter 2: EKG THEORY

EKG INTERPRETATION MADE EASY

Criterias	Sinus Bradycardia	Sinus Tachycardia	Sinus Arrhythmia	Sinus Pause/Arrest	Sinus Atrial Block
P wave	Present	Present	Present	Present	Present
QRS Duration	Normal	Normal	Normal	Normal	Normal
P-R Interval	Normal	Normal	Normal	Normal	Normal
Rhythm	Regular	Regular	Irregular	Irregular	Irregular
Rate	< 60	>100	Varies 60-100	Varies(slow) Pause Present	Varies(slow) Beat Absent

TABLE 2.10

Criterias	Wandering Atrial Pacemaker	Premature Atrial Contraction	Atrial Tachycardia	Atrial Flutter	Atrial Fibrillation
P wave	Different Shapes	Different Shapes	Varies in Shapes	Saw-tooth Appearance	Chaotic Wave
QRS Duration	Normal	Normal	Normal	Normal	Normal
PR Interval	Varies	Varies PAC present	Short	Varies	None
Rhythm	Irregular	Irregular	Regular	Regular to Varies	Irregular
Rate	Normal	Varies 60-100	> 100	Atrial Fast Ventricular Slow	Atrial Fast Ventricular Slow

TABLE 2.11

Criterias	Junctional Rhythm	Accelerated Junctional Rhythm	Junctional Tachycardia	Junctional Escape Beat	Premature Junctional Contraction
P wave	Inverted, Buried, or Absent	Inverted, Buried, or Absent	Inverted, Buried, or Absent	Inverted, Buried, or Absent	Inverted, Buried, or Absent
QRS Duration	Normal	Normal	Normal	Normal	Normal
P-R Interval	Short or Absent	Short or Absent	Short or Absent	Short or Absent	Shorter, Buried, or Absent
Rhythm	Regular	Regular	Regular	Irregular when Escape Beat	Irregular when PJC
Rate	<60	60 - 100	>100	Depend on underlying rhythm	Depend on underlying rhythm

TABLE 2.12

Criterias	Supra Ventricular Tachycardia	Idio Ventricular Rhythm	Premature Ventricular Contraction	Ventricular Tachycardia	Ventricular Fibrillation
P wave	Buried with "T" Difficult to identify	Absent	Unable to identify when PVC occurs	Absent	None
QRS Duration	Usually Normal	Wide	Wide when PVC occurs	Wide	None
P-R Interval	Unable to measure	None	None when PVC occurs	None	None
Rhythm	Regular	Regular	Irregular	Regular	None
Rate	>100	<60	Depend on underlying rhythm	>100	Cannot determine

TABLE 2.13

Criterias	First Degree Block	Second Degree Block Type I	Second Degree Block Type II	Third Degree Block	Bundle Branch Block
P wave	Present	Present	Present	Present	Present
QRS Duration	Normal	Normal	Wide	Normal or Wide	Wide
P-R Interval	Prolonged	Widening Progressively with a missing QRS	Normal to Prolong	Varies	Normal
Rhythm	Regular	Irregular	Regular: Atrial Irregular: Ventricular	Independent Atria/Ventricle	Regular or Irregular
Rate	Varies	Varies	Atrial Normal Ventricular Slow	Atrial Normal Ventricular Slow	Varies

TABLE 2.14

Criterias	Torsade De Pointes	Asystole
P wave	N/A	N/A
QRS Duration	N/A	N/A
P-R Interval	N/A	N/A
Rhythm	Irregular	N/A
Rate	Fast	N/A

TABLE 2.15

Criterias	Atrial Single Chamber Pacemaker	Ventricular Single Chamber Pacemaker	Atrial & Ventricular Dual Chamber Pacemaker
P wave	Present	Absent	Present
QRS Duration	Normal	Wide	Wide
P-R Interval	Normal	N/A	N/A
Spike	Before P wave	Before Q wave	1 Before P wave 1 Before Q wave
Rate	Varies	Varies	Varies

TABLE 2.16

LEAD AND VIEW

LEAD I Lateral	aVR	V1 Septal	V4 Anterior
LEAD II Inferior	aVL Lateral	V2 Septal	V5 Lateral
LEAD III Inferior	aVF Inferior	V3 Anterior	V6 Lateral

TABLE 2.17

What is Axis deviation in EKG?

This is when the heart rotates from its axis

Right Side Axis Deviation	Left Side Axis Deviation
S wave greater than R wave in	S wave greater than R wave in
LEAD I	**LEAD II**

Atrial Hypertrophy

Biphasic P wave

Right Atrial Hypertrophy	Left Atrial Hypertrophy
Component 1 Large	Component 1 Small
Component 2 Smaller	Component 2 Wide

What is pathological Q WAVE

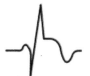

Pathological Q Wave Infarction

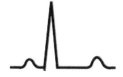

Normal Q Wave

What is the placement of V7 electrode

V7
Posterior Axillary Line on Left Side Lateral to V6

V7R
Posterior Axillary Line on Right Side Lateral to V6R

What is Holter Monitoring

- It is a form of EKG device in which the patients cardiac activities are monitored for 24 to 48 hours.

- It is a non-invasive procedure.

- It includes 5 or 7 electrodes.

- It records the cardiac activity for 24 to 48 hours (pre-recorded event).

- Skin preparation should be done before electrode placement.

- Normal activities can be done while the device is attached to the body during the 24 to 48hr period.

Indications

1. Evaluation of symptoms suggesting arrhythmia or myocardial ischemia.

2. Evaluation of EKG documenting therapeutic interventions in individual patients or groups of patients.

3. Evaluation of patients for ST segment changes.

4. Evaluation of a patient's response after resuming occupational or recreational activities (e.g., after M.I. or cardiac surgery.)

5. Clinical and epidemiological research studies.

6. Evaluation of patients with pacemakers.

7. Reporting of time and frequency domain heart rate variability.

8. Reporting of QT Interval.

Points to consider:

1. Do not splash water on holter monitoring device or electrodes.

2. Do not store the device in a humid or area of sunlight.

3. Do not drop the device.

4. Do not remove the batteries while the monitor is recording activity.

Electrode sites should be dry and not wet at all times to avoid detachment of electrodes from the skin surface.

Telemetry

Telemetry is a form of EKG device in which the electrodes are placed on the patient's chest and connected to the transmitter, this transmitter than turns the signals in waves, these waves are picked up by the receiver at the central monitoring unit location which shows the waves in the form of an EKG recording.

Make sure to contact the central monitoring unit location to check whether the central monitoring unit is receiving the signals of the new patient for monitoring.

Event Monitor

Event monitor is an EKG device which records the electrical activity of the heart only when the symptom arises.

Different types of event monitor:

Type 1. In some monitors, patients have to turn on the device when the symptom is felt.

Type 2. In some monitors, the monitor automatically detects the abnormal rhythm and switches on.

ST SEGMENT CHANGES

ST Segment Elevation	ST Segment Depression

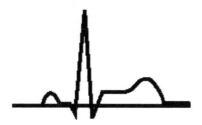

ST Segment above the baseline	ST Segment below the baseline

END OF CHAPTER REVIEW

1. Electrocardiography is the procedure by which _Electrical_ activities of the heart are recorded.

2. The spread of excitation throughout the myocardium cells produces electrical potential, this potential causes a current flow, which acts as a _Volume Conductor_

3. _Electrocardiograph_ is the instrument (machine) by which electrical activities of the heart are recorded.

4. Electrocardiogram (EKG or ECG) is the _graphical Representation_ of electrical activities of the heart.

5. Which of the following is not a use of ekg?

    a) _____ To determine heart rate

    b) _____ To determine heart rhythm

    c) _✓_ To obtain a radiographic image

    d) _____ To determine coronary artery disease

6. _Duration (TIME)_ of EKG waves is plotted horizontally on X-axis.

7. *On X-axis*

    1 mm = _0.04_ second

    _5_ mm = 0.20 second

8. _Amplitude_ of EKG waves is plotted vertically on Y-axis.

9. *On Y-axis*

    _1_ mm = 0.1 mV

    5 mm = _0.5_ mV

10. Speed of the paper during recording is fixed at _25_ mm/second. If heart rate is very high, speed of the paper is changed to _50_ mm/second.

11. EKG is recorded in 12 leads, which are generally classified into two categories _bipolar_ leads & _unipolar_ leads

12. *Bipolar Limb leads* are otherwise known as standard limb leads (SLL).

13. Standard limb leads are of three types _Limb lead 1_, _Limb lead 2_ & _Limb lead 3_

14. _limb lead 1_ is generated by connecting right arm and left arm. Right arm is connected to the _positive_ terminal of the EKG unit and the left arm is connected to the _Negative_ terminal.

15. _limb lead 2_ is generated by connecting right arm and left leg. Right arm is connected to the _positive_ terminal of the EKG unit and the left leg is connected to the _Negative_ terminal.

16. _Limb lead 3_ is generated by connecting left arm and left leg. Left arm is connected to the _positive_ terminal of the EKG unit and the left leg is connected to the _Negative_ terminal.

17. Standard Limb Leads are of three types:

   a. Limb Lead I   = LA (_positive_ ELECTRODE) + _RA_ (NEGATIVE ELECTRODE)

   b. Limb Lead II = LL (_positive_ ELECTRODE) + _RA_ (NEGATIVE ELECTRODE)

   c. Limb Lead III = _LL_ (POSITIVE ELECTRODE) + LA (_Negative_ ELECTRODE)

18. Unipolar limb leads are also called _Augmented_ limb leads.

19. Unipolar limb leads are of three types: _AVL_ , _AVR_ & _AVF_

20. aVR lead : Active electrode is directed towards the _Right_ arm.

21. _aVL_ lead : Active electrode is directed towards the left arm.

22. aVF lead : Active electrode is directed towards the _Left_ leg.

23. Chest leads are denoted as 'V' leads or _precordial_ chest leads.

24. Label the electrode placements

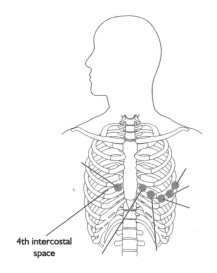

4th intercostal
space

**A. Standard chest lead
placement**

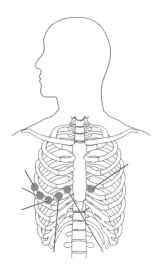

**B. Right sided chest
lead placement**

25. Position of chest leads:

    a) V1 : Over ___4___th intercostal space near __Right__ sternal margin

    b) V2 : Over ___4___th intercostal space near __Left__ sternal margin

    c) V3 : In between ___V2___ and ___V4___

    d) V4 : Over left ___5___th intercostal space on the mid clavicular line

    e) V5 : Over left ___5___th intercostal space on the _Anterior_ axillary line

    f) V6 : Over left ___5___th intercostal space on the _Mid_ axillary line.

26. __P___ wave is a first positive wave seen in the EKG. It is also called atrial complex wave.

27. __P___ wave is produced due to the _dsploRatioN_ of atria of the heart.

Chapter 2: EKG THEORY

28. ___P___ wave is normally positive & upright in leads I, II, aVF, V4, V5 and V6. It is normally negative (inverted) in __AVR__.

29. 'QRS' complex is the __VENTRICULAR COMPLEX__

30. ___Q___ wave is a negative wave

31. 'QRS' complex is due to __depolarization__ of ventricular chambers of the heart.

32. 'Q' wave is due to the depolarization (basal portion) of __INTER VENTRICULAR SEPTUM__

33. 'S' wave represents the depolarization of basal portion of __VENTRICULAR__ musculature.

34. Normal duration of 'QRS' complex is between 0.06 and __0.10__ second.

35. 'T' wave is due to the repolarization (relaxation) of __VENTRICULAR__ muscles.

36. 'T' wave is normally positive in leads I, II and V__5__ and V __6__

37. 'U' wave is supposed to be due to repolarization of __Papillary Muscles__ or __Purkinje Fibers__.

38. 'P-R' interval is the interval from the start of ___P___ wave and __End__ of 'Q' wave.

39. 'P-R' interval signifies the conduction of impulses through __AV__ node.

40. 'P' wave represents the __Atrial__ depolarization.

41. Normal duration of 'P-R interval' varies between __0.12__ and __0.20__ second.

42. 'Q-T' interval is the interval from the __Start__ of the 'Q' wave to the __End__ of 'T' wave.

43. 'Q-T' interval indicates the ventricular __depolarization__ and ventricular __Repolarization__

44. 'S-T' segment is the interval between the end of the '_S_' wave and the onset of '_T_' wave.

45. __Q.T__ interval signifies the duration of one cardiac cycle.

46. IDENTIFY GRAPH: Normal Sinus Rhythm **HR:** 71

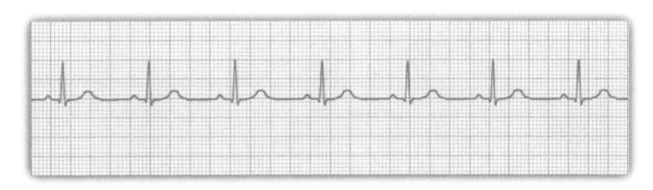

47. IDENTIFY GRAPH: Sinus Bradycardia **HR:** 50

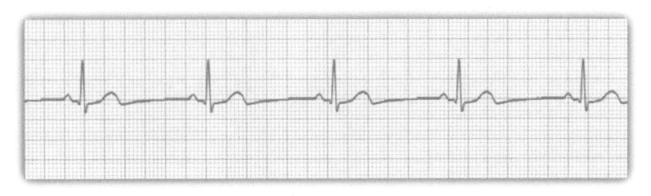

48. IDENTIFY GRAPH: Sinus Tachycardia **HR:** 150

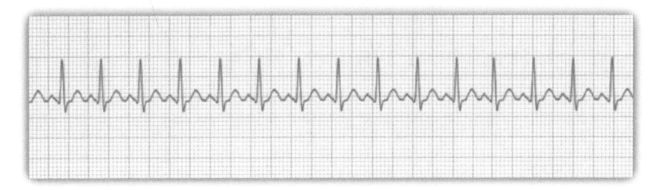

49.IDENTIFY GRAPH: *Sinus Arrhythmia*   **HR:** 50

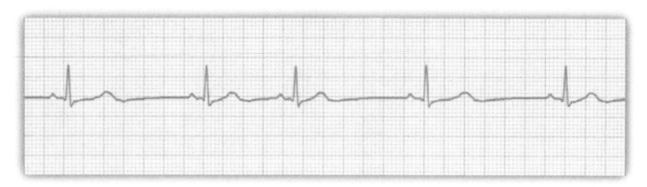

50.IDENTIFY GRAPH: *Sino-Atrial Block*   **HR:** 70

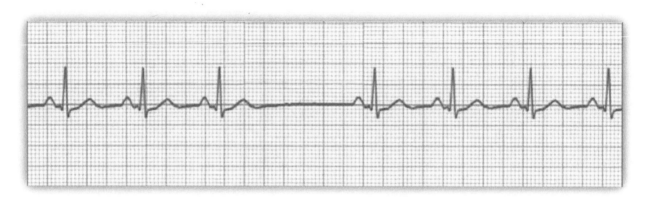

51.IDENTIFY GRAPH: *Premature Atrial Contraction* **HR:** 80

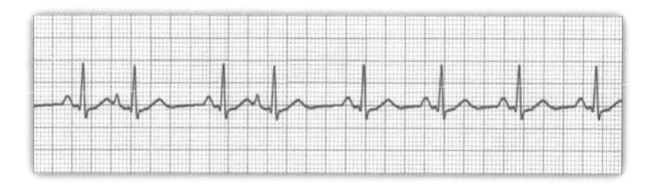

52.IDENTIFY GRAPH: Atrial Flutter   **HR:** 90

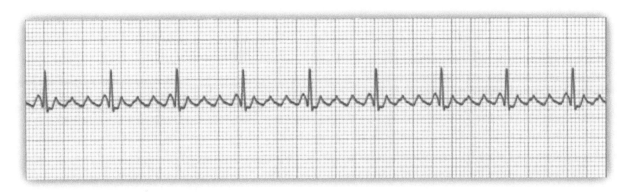

53.IDENTIFY GRAPH: Atrial Fibrillation   **HR:** 100

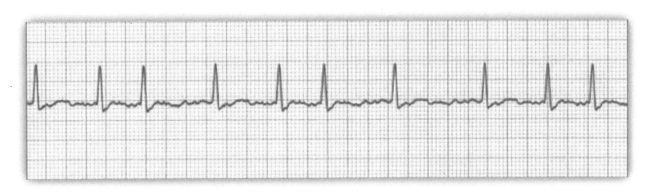

54.IDENTIFY GRAPH: SuperVentricular Tachycardia   **HR:** 190

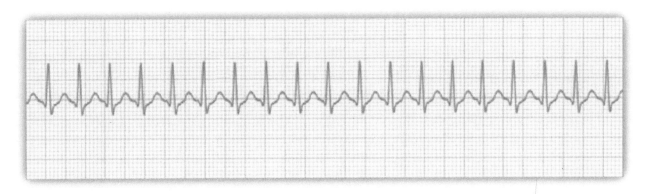

55.IDENTIFY GRAPH: *first degree block* **HR:** 70

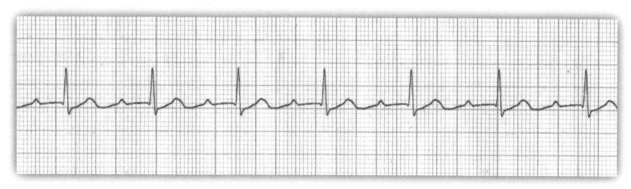

56.IDENTIFY GRAPH: Second degree block Type 2 **HR:** 40

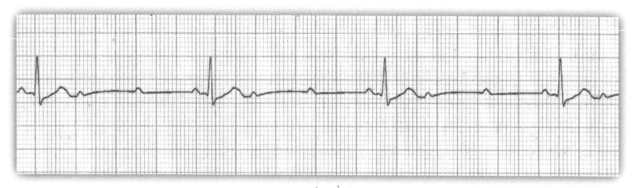

complete

57.IDENTIFY GRAPH: Third degree Block **HR:** 30

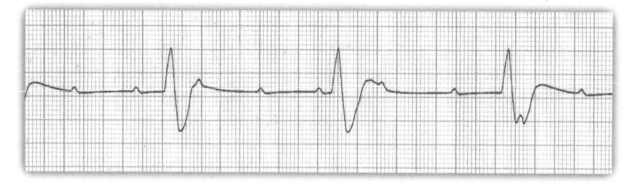

58.IDENTIFY GRAPH: Idioventricular Rhythm **HR:** 30

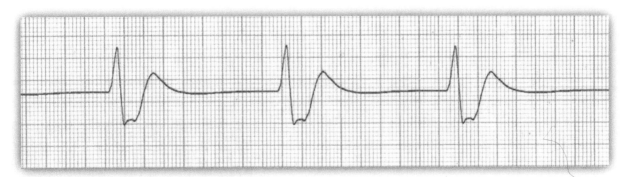

59.IDENTIFY GRAPH: Ventricular Fibrillation **HR:**

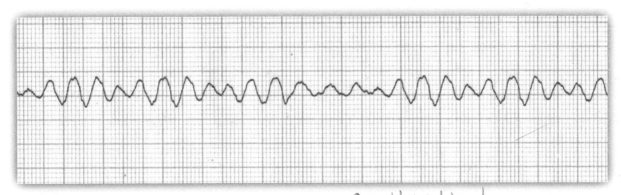

contration

60.IDENTIFY GRAPH: Premature Ventricular **HR:** 70

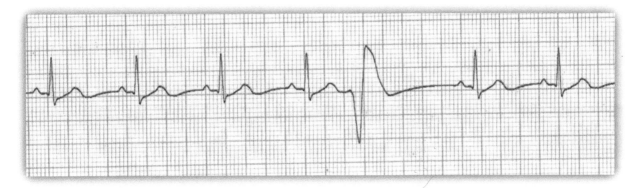

CHAPTER 3

ELECTROCARDIOGRAPHY CLINICAL

INDICATIONS & CONTRAINDICATIONS OF EKG

Few indications for reporting an electrocardiogram (EKG)

- Patients with chest pain
- Dizziness undetermined
- Monitoring cardiovascular disease
- Diagnosis or Prognosis & follow up of cardiovascular disease
- Effect of medication
- Pre-operative assessment workup for surgery
- Risk analysis for cardiac diseases
- Routine examination of non-cardiac patients

Few contraindications for an electrocardiogram (EKG)

- Patients not willing to consent
- Patient with abusive or mentally unstable or uncooperative behavior making it difficult for the procedure to take place
- Unable to place electrodes on the proper areas of the body surface due to trauma, skin burns or skin conditions which limits the placement of electrodes.

The diagnostic information of an EKG can be divided into three classifications:

- **C**onduction Abnormalities (rhythm, improper functioning of pacemakers)
- **A**natomical Abnormalities (injury, ischemia, infarction, heart enlargement, dextrocardia)
- **P**hysiological Abnormalities (cardiac cycle anomaly)

Remember the word **CAP**

IS THE EKG ACCURATE?

It is crucial to remember that an EKG is never hundred percent accurate, the reason being many factors such as artifacts, improper training, casual approach towards electrode application, standard procedures not being followed appropriately.

Adhering to the standard protocol & principle for performing the procedure may limit the inaccuracy, thereby improving the process of electrocardiography.

The surface anatomy for electrode placement in electrocardiography can be divided into two parts

1. **Surface Anatomy of Limbs for EKG Electrode Placements**

2. **Surface Anatomy of Thorax for EKG Electrode Placements**

SURFACE ANATOMY OF LIMBS FOR EKG ELECTRODE PLACEMENTS:

The limb anatomy consist of the

Upper two limbs also called upper two extremities

- Order from Shoulder to Finger Tips are as follows: ***Proximal to Distal***
- Shoulder Joint, Humerus, Elbow Joint, Radius, Ulna, Carpals, Metacarpals, Phalanges

Lower two limbs also called lower two extremities:

- Order from Hip to Toe Tip are as follows: ***Proximal to Distal***
- Hip Joint, Femur, Knee Joint, Patella, Tibia, Fibula, Tarsals, Metatarsals, Phalanges
  Note: The bony prominence proximal to the ankle joint medially (medial malleolus) and laterally (lateral malleolus) are lower ends of tibia and fibula respectively

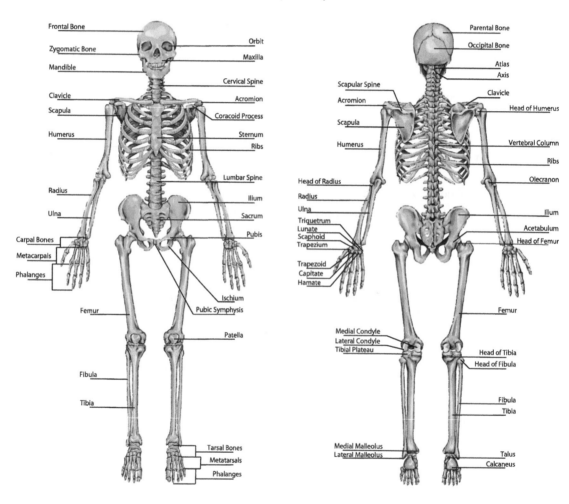

FIGURE 3.1

SURFACE ANATOMY OF THORAX FOR EKG ELECTRODE PLACEMENTS:

The thorax anatomy consists of:

- Sternum, Costal Cartilage, Ribs, Intercostal Space, Intercostal Muscles and Vertebrae.

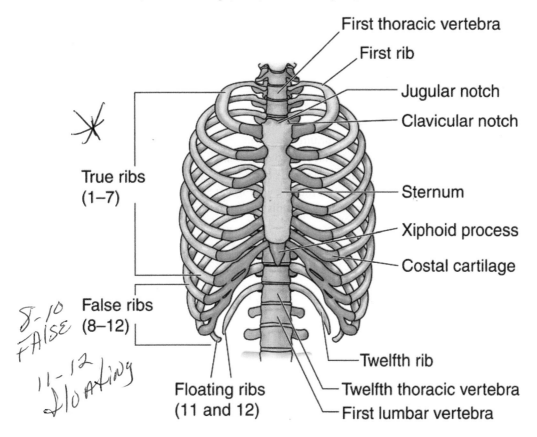

FIGURE 3.2

Orientation of Thorax	Structures
Anterior View (Front)	Sternum, Costal Cartilages, Ribs, Intercostal Space, Intercostal Muscles
Lateral View (Side)	Ribs, Intercostal Space, Intercostal Muscles
Posterior View (Back)	Ribs, Intercostal Space, Intercostal Muscles, Vertebrae

Note: In the posterior view of the thorax, scapula bone (triangular shaped bone) lies over the ribs.

Sternum bone is located centrally and in front of the thorax and is further divided into three parts:

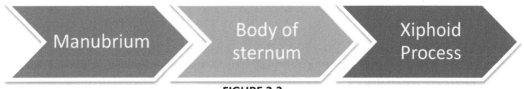

FIGURE 3.3

Note: Connection between **Manubrium** & **Body of Sternum** is called the **Angle of Louis** also known as **Sternal Angle,** this is where the 2nd pair of costal cartilages is attached, while palpating for the intercostal space moving distally from the 2nd pair of costal cartilage will lead to finding of the 2nd intercostal space.

The sternal angle can be easily palpated except in individuals with well developed muscles or obesity.

- o Summary Hint: The second set of ribs is attached to the sternal angle laterally, below which is the 2nd intercostal space **(ICS)**.

WOODEN STICK TECHNIQUE TO FIND THE STERNAL ANGLE

Method of finding the 2nd Intercostal Space

Step 1. Get two wooden sticks used for collecting swab samples.

Step 2. Place one wooden stick along the body of the sternum.

Step 3. Place another wooden stick along the manubrium.

Step 4. Make sure both the wooden sticks are in their respective positions.

Step 5. Look for the point where both the wooden sticks cross each other, the point of the sticks crossing each other is the sternal angle also known as angle of Louis, moving your fingers laterally to this sternal angle will lead you to the 2nd costal cartilage (2nd pair of rib), moving fingers distally from this location (2nd pair of ribs) will lead to a space (2nd intercostal space).

Left Mid-Clavicular Line & Anterior Axillary Line

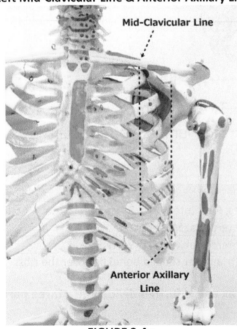

FIGURE 3.4a

Mid-Axillary Line

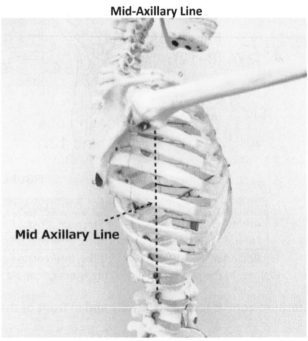

FIGURE 3.4b

Hints

- Do not use nipples as a reference location for 4th intercostal space in individuals with hypertrophied muscles, obesity or breast tissues.
- Nipples should not be used as a reference point.
- Nipples are not always located on the mid-clavicular line.

SPECIAL CONSIDERATION FOR ANATOMICAL & PATHOLOGICAL CHANGES (ANATOMY OF THE THORAX)

Pectus Excavatum (Concave depression of the thorax)

- Placement of V1 & V2 becomes difficult due to the depression of the anterior thorax centrally.

Pectus Carinatum (Convex elevation or protruding of the thorax due to over growth of costal cartilages)

- Placement of V1-V6 becomes difficult due to the protrusion of the anterior thorax.

Obesity

- Subcutaneous fat can make it hard to palpate the surface anatomy.

Hypertrophic Muscles

- Muscle bulk can make it difficult to palpate the surface anatomy for electrode placement.(*due to the muscle size*)

Trauma or Surgery

- Recent surgeries can make it difficult to palpate the skin surface, also the symmetry of the ribs may be compromised (asymmetrical) post surgery, consideration and care must be taken in these cases to understand the changes.

Breast Augmentation

- Difficulty for electrode placement may vary based on the size of augmentation.

Mastectomy

- Skin condition post mastectomy must be taken into consideration prior to placement of electrodes.

PATIENT POSITIONING FOR PROPER ELECTRODE PLACEMENTS

Supine position is the most appropriate position in which the patient should be positioned for an EKG procedure, The person performing the procedure should ensure that when the patient is in this position the arms and legs of the patient should be relaxed, if in any case the muscles of the lower limb are not relaxed try placing a pillow under the patient's knees which leads to a release of tension in the lower extremities due to flexion of the knees. One pillow should be placed under the patient's head for support and comfort.

If for medical reasons the standard patient position (supine position) cannot be achieved position the patient in a semi-fowler position. (*A position achieved by placing the patient midway between supine and sitting position*)

PROCEED TOWARDS THE STANDARD ELECTRODE PLACEMENT

While placing electrodes on a patient make sure that each and every electrode is placed on the most appropriate location as per the standard protocol for an electrocardiogram, inappropriate placement of electrodes on the patient may lead to inaccurate results or misdiagnosis. If the electrodes are not placed appropriately, this may lead to changes in the PQRST waves, QRS complex, ST segment, PR interval, or QT interval.

PLACEMENT FOR STANDARD LIMB ELECTRODES (SLE)

- **Right Arm** electrode can be placed **proximal** to the **Right Wrist.**
- **Left Arm** electrode can be placed **proximal** to the **Left Wrist.**
- **Right Leg** electrode can be placed **proximal** to the **Right Ankle.**
- **Left Leg** electrode can be placed **proximal** to the **Left Ankle.**

Notes

- Avoid placing standard limb electrodes on bony prominences as this may compromise the proper contact of the electrodes on the patient's skin.
- Studies have shown that moving the electrodes more proximally from the standard positions can lead to changes in the EKG waveforms.
- Have your patient completely relaxed before placing the limb electrodes to eliminate the muscle artifacts caused by the patient movements after placement of the limb electrodes.
- The wrist joint and the ankle joint should be visible to the person applying electrodes.
- Have the patient remove any type of restrictive accessories from the wrist and ankle if it affects the electrode placements. (make sure the accessories are nonmedical and nonreligious)
- Take patient's permission before exposing and touching any part of the patient's body.

PLACEMENT FOR STANDARD CHEST ELECTRODES

(Pre-cordial electrodes or chest electrodes)

V1 : 4th intercostal space on the right of the sternal border

V2 : 4th intercostal space on the left of the sternal border

V3 : Midway between V2 & V4

V4 : 5th intercostal space on the left mid-clavicular line

V5 : In line with V4 on the left anterior axillary line

V6 : In line with V5 on the left mid-axillary line

Note: Never place the chest electrodes by guessing their locations because thoracic anatomy changes from individual to individual, placing the electrodes by guessing may lead to inaccurate results and misdiagnosis.

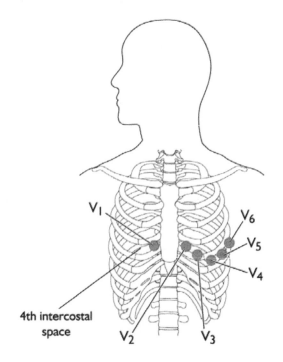

Standard chest lead placement

FIGURE 3.5

Chapter 3: EKG CLINICAL

PRACTICALLY APPLYING THE ELECTRODES CAN BE DONE IN THE FOLLOWING STEPWISE MANNER

How to locate V1 Electrode Placement?

Locate the angle of louis or sternal angle, once found move laterally towards the right to palpate the 2nd rib, slide over the 2nd rib distally into the 2nd inter-costal space further slide over the 3rd rib distally into the 3rd intercostal space, proceed to slide over the 4th rib distally into the 4th inter-costal space, Place the V1 electrode in the 4th intercostal space on the right of the sternum.

How to locate V2 & V4 Electrode Placement?

Repeat the above steps on the left side for V2 electrode placement in the 4th intercostal space on the left side. Slide over the 5th rib distally into the 5th inter-costal space. Once the 5th intercostal space in located, look for the mid-clavicular line bisecting perpendicularly over the 5th intercostal space, once located place the V4 electrode on the location.

How to locate V3 Electrode Placement?

Place V3 electrode midway between V2 & V4.

How to locate V5 Electrode Placement?

From the V4 intercostal space move fingers laterally to a point on the anterior axillary line, place the V5 electrode at this location, anterior axillary line can be found by placing the patients arm close to the body and looking for the crease of the skin at the front of the patients armpit.

How to locate V6 Electrode Placement?

From V5 electrode placement move fingers laterally (horizontally) to a point where the mid-axillary line bisects, once found place the V6 electrode.

Hint

In females, while placing the electrodes underneath the breast tissue, the most appropriate technique used would be, wearing gloves and lifting the breast tissue using the back of the hand to push the breast tissue gently upwards, Always avoid using fingers to hold the breast tissue during electrode placement. If the patient is willing to help in lifting the breast tissue in an upward direction for electrode placement allow the patient to do so.

SPECIAL CONSIDERATIONS SHOULD BE MADE WHILE PERFORMING AN ELECTROCARDIOGRAM ON:

Amputated Extremity

The standard limb electrodes shall be placed as distally as possible for performing the procedure.

Breast Tissue

- **Large breast tissue**

  If the patient is willing to help in lifting up their own breast tissue, respect their decision as most females are comfortable doing it especially when the procedure in being performed by a male. Make sure that the breast tissue is placed in an upward position until the electrode placement is complete for that specific electrode.

- **Augmented breast tissue**

  The enhanced breast tissues may extend upto the 5th intercostal space which makes it difficult to lift and palpate the breast tissue with the back of the hand for the placement of V4, also the breast tissue may cover the 4th intercostal space near the sternal border making it difficult to place the V1 & V2, another issue is the scar underneath the breast tissue, hence care should be taken that the electrodes should not be placed on the scar tissue, reason being scar tissues can create high skin impedance.

Condition of the skin

- **Skin disorder**

  Different skin conditions may lead to derangement of skin integrity causing changes in skin impedance.

- **Burns**

  Depending on the degree and type of burn, the electrode placement may become difficult, as the skin may be painful to touch due to the tissue damage.

Heart on the right side (Dextrocardiac)

Mirror image of normal 12 lead EKG electrode placements shall be followed in this case.

Critical thinking!

Does it matter if the limb electrodes are placed on any location on the limb?

Note: This placement will change the waveforms and voltage conduction from electrodes

Your Comments:

_____

_____

_____

_____

_____

Is it appropriate to place the arm electrodes on upper arm(near shoulder joint) and leg electrodes on the upper leg (near hip joint) or should the arm electrodes be placed at the lower arm just proximal to the wrist and leg electrodes on lower leg just proximal to the ankle joint?

Your Comments:

_____

_____

_____

_____

_____

Is it true that V4, V5, V6, are in the 5th intercostal space or just in line with each other?

Your Comments:

_____

_____

_____

_____

_____

Is it fine if the electrodes are placed slightly away from their standard location?

Your Comments:

_____

_____

_____

_____

_____

How to get an artifact free EKG?

Your Comments:

_____

_____

_____

_____

_____

What happens to the R waves if the V1 & V2 electrodes are placed higher up from their standard electrode locations?

Your Comments:

_____

_____

_____

SKIN IMPEDANCE

Skin impedance is the resistance against the electrical conduction from the skin surface, lowering the skin impedance is a crucial step in obtaining an artifact free EKG recording.

To reduce the skin impedance, appropriate time should be spend for skin preparation before the placement of the electrodes on the patient's skin.

SKIN PREPARATION PROCESS

Some causes of high skin impedance:

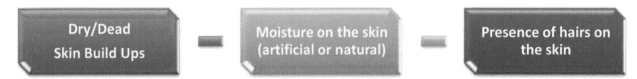

Dry/Dead Skin Build Ups — Moisture on the skin (artificial or natural) — Presence of hairs on the skin

Methods of skin preparation

Oily & Greasy Skin

- Normal oily skin should be cleansed with a mild soap solution, if the skin has access moisture an alcohol based cleansers can be used to clean the surface of the skin, remember to completely let the alcohol evaporate from the surface of the skin before applying or placing the electrode on the cleansed area for better adhesion between the electrode and the skin surface. Another precaution that should be taken into consideration is of letting the alcohol dry on the surface of the skin which is already dry, this may lead to high skin impedance and low quality diagnostic EKG, Hence special precautions should be taken if the patient has dry skin.

- Abrading the skin lightly with disposable dry gauze, or by using special fine sand disposable papers used for abrading skin if access moisture or dry skin build up is found to be present on the surface of the skin which cannot be cleaned by the regular alcohol pad. Care should be taken while performing this abrasion technique. The skin should not be visibly scratched, it should just turn light pink in color. Practicing this technique during the training can help to perform better in real life situations. The most important part of the technique is the application of pressure during the abrasion process. Remember the pressure should be as light as possible taking into consideration the condition of the patient's skin.

Note: *Skin preparation is one of the least focused technique when performing EKG and is often not taken seriously leading to high skin impedance and low skin conduction which eventually results in a low quality diagnostic EKG.*

Hair on the skin

If the patient has hair on the location were the electrodes are to be placed according to the standard placement for respective standard electrodes. Removing the hair from the location would be the appropriate step that should be practiced.

If the electrodes are applied to the surface of the patient's skin without removing the hairs, it may lead to impartial or incomplete adhesion of the electrodes resulting in improper conduction and potential artifact.

When removing hair from the skin surface use professional hair clippers. Do not remove the hair in a horizontal direction (across the patient's chest) when using the hair clippers, but rather in the direction of the hair growth. This causes less irritation to the patients skin during and after the procedure. After removing the hairs the patient's skin should be cleansed with a mild soap solution or alcohol pad depending on the condition of the skin.

Hint

Care should be taken during skin preparation on conditions like

- Burns
- Eczema
- Fungal infection on the skin
- Open wounds
- Scar or keloid tissue
- Or any other skin condition that may cause skin injury due to the skin preparation process

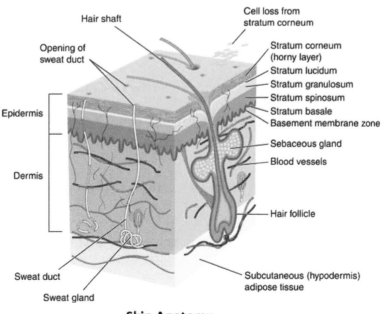

Skin Anatomy

EKG ELECTRODES

The function of the electrodes is to conduct the electrical activity of the heart from the surface of the skin and bring it to the EKG recording unit via the EKG cables connected to each electrode.

Two types of EKG electrodes are:

DISPOSABLE ELECTRODES:

Advantages

- is readily available
- no need to spend time for disinfecting the electrodes after use
- available in different shapes and sizes
- easy to apply and remove from the surface of the skin
- less chances of cross infection from patient to patient

Disadvantages

- cannot be reused
- comes with an expiration date after which it cannot be used
- should be stored by using the proper technique to maintain the quality of the electrodes as per manufacturer instructions

NON-DISPOSABLE ELECTRODES:

Advantages

- can be reused

Disadvantages

- expensive
- more chances of cross infection from patient to patient
- has to be disinfected after every use
- application may not be easy

Applying and removing the electrodes from the patient's skin should be done in a proper way.

To apply the electrodes on the patient's skin depending on the type of electrodes used

- The electrode should be in firm contact with the patient's skin.

To remove the electrodes from the patient's skin

- Care should be taken to avoid pulling of the skin when trying to peel off the electrodes, be gentle when peeling off the electrodes.

Note: *Remember to clean the patient's skin after the removal of the electrodes, as many electrodes leave residue on the patient's skin which may cause skin irritation.*

Direction of electrode placement

Applying electrodes in any direction will lead to uneven tension of wires resulting in an artifact. When applying electrodes on the patient's skin place the right arm, left arm, V1 to V6 electrodes wires directed towards the feet, and the right leg and left leg electrode wires directed towards the head of the patient, this may cause less pulling of the wires in different directions.

Make sure that the electrodes are properly connected to the alligator-clips, as improper connection between the electrode and alligator-clips will result in incomplete or no transmission of electrical activity from the skin to the EKG unit.

ADDITIONAL ILLUSTRATIONS

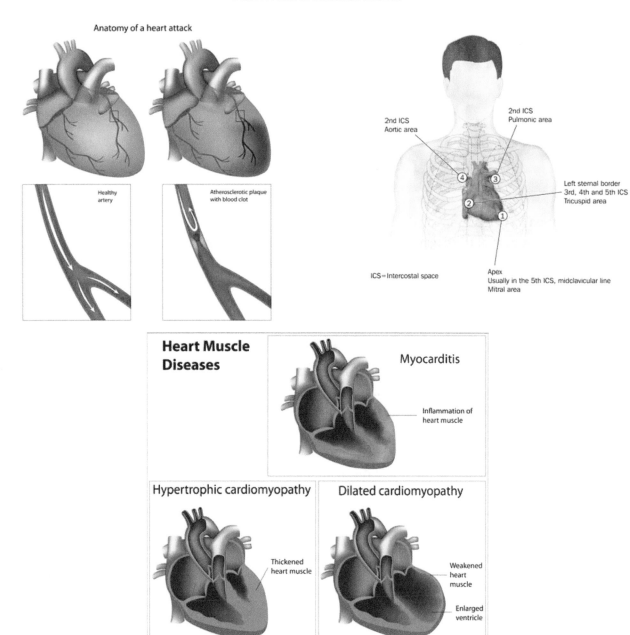

Anatomy of a heart attack

Healthy artery

Atherosclerotic plaque with blood clot

2nd ICS Aortic area

2nd ICS Pulmonic area

Left sternal border 3rd, 4th and 5th ICS Tricuspid area

ICS = Intercostal space

Apex Usually in the 5th ICS, midclavicular line Mitral area

Heart Muscle Diseases

Myocarditis

Inflammation of heart muscle

Hypertrophic cardiomyopathy

Thickened heart muscle

Dilated cardiomyopathy

Weakened heart muscle

Enlarged ventricle

EQUIPMENTS SHOULD BE CHECKED BEFORE ITS USE

Sensitivity and Gain

Is a response of the EKG unit to a specific applied voltage, according to the standard.

> 1mv (milli-volt) will cause a 10mm (millimeter) deflection.

Standardization & Calibration

Setting the EKG unit to record the standard is called as standardization or calibration

The standard calibration signals should be 10mm high and 5mm wide.

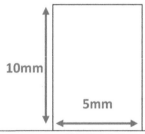

10mm

5mm

FIGURE 3.6

The calibration mark representing the sensitivity or gain of the EKG machine is printed usually on the left-hand side of the page at the beginning of each line of EKG and should be two large squares 10mm in height this means that for every milli-volt measured from the patient, a deflection of 10mm will be recorded on the trace. For the purpose of EKG recording the terms gain and sensitivity are interchangeable.

When performing an EKG:

- When the waves are bigger in size and are being deflected beyond the EKG graph paper, lower the sensitivity control on the gain, this change will cause the waves to record half the size of the impulse leading to proper wave recording on the EKG paper.

- When the waves are small in size, increase the sensitivity control on the gain, this change will cause the waves to record double the size of the impulse leading to proper wave recording on the EKG paper.

  Note: *Make sure to document the change in the gain so that the practitioner is aware about the changes. Once done bring the gain back to normal.*

PAPER SPEED

Setting the paper speed

Standard paper speed is 25mm/sec

This paper speed denotes that the EKG paper prints at a speed of 25mm per second from the EKG unit.

Setting the paper speed of 50mm/sec

- For pediatric EKG monitoring
- For adults with tachycardia

The speed change to 50mm/sec helps in differentiating whether the tachycardia is atrial or ventricular.

When the speed is set at 50mm/sec the graph may look like

- Bradycardia
- Prolong PR
- Prolong QRS
- Prolong QT

Note: *It is very important to document the speed at which the graph was recorded.*

EKG FILTERS

What are EKG filters?

Filter is a feature in the EKG unit with which the unwanted signals are filtered out leading to a true and clear graphical representation of the electrical activity of the heart on the EKG paper.

Some reasons for using the EKG filter for the procedures would be

1. To avoid wandering baseline due to
   a. sweating
   b. patient movement
   c. breathing movement of chest
2. To avoid electromagnetic interference
3. To avoid muscle noise
4. To avoid noise from the instrument or unit
5. To avoid electrode contact noise (loose electrode or motion artifact)

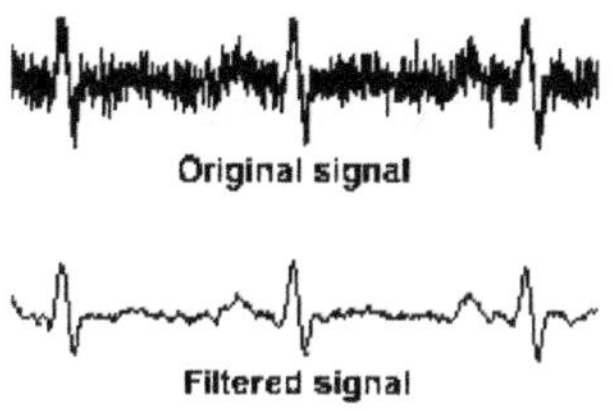

Original signal

Filtered signal

FIGURE 3.7

Diagnostics Filter Types:

- Low pass filtering with a cut off frequency
- High pass filtering with a cut off frequency

EQUIPMENT AND SUPPLIES LIST FOR EKG

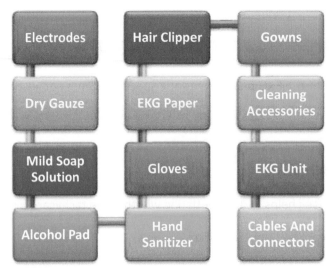

FIGURE 3.8

Points to consider

- Prepare the patient for recording EKG by having good communication with the patient prior to the procedure as this may lead to a decrease in stress and anxiety of the patient.
- Identify the patient
  - Check patients his or her first and last name, date of birth in an outpatient setting.
  - Check patients his or her first and last name, date of birth and patient ID number in a inpatient setting.
- Explain the patient that he or she has been referred for an EKG.
- Request the patient to be still while the EKG procedure is in process.
- Before printing the EKG make sure to check for the leads on the LCD monitor of the EKG unit.
- After the procedure, if the EKG shows abnormality that would require attention it should be reported immediately to the supervising practitioner.

An EKG procedure should

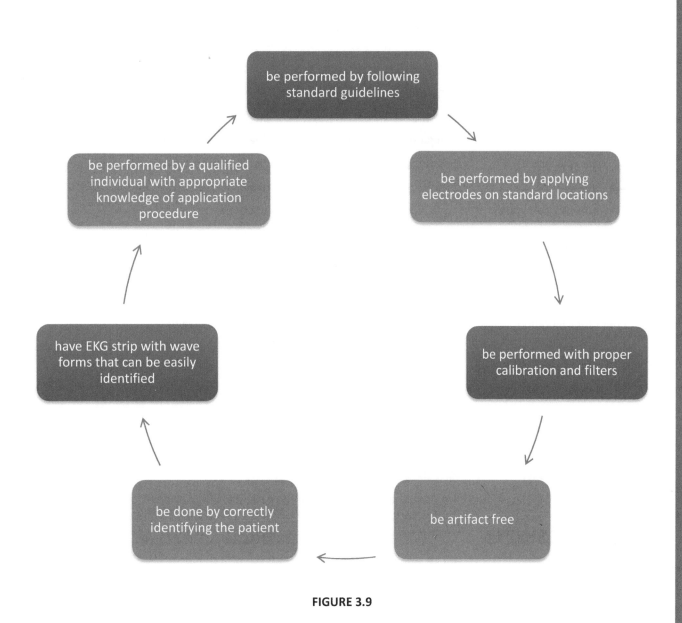

FIGURE 3.9

3.1. Table

OBJECTIVES	RATIONALE
EKG equipment	Equipment's must be ready to use for the procedure to take place. (PS)
Introduce yourself	This assures the patient. (PBR)
Confirming patients identity	Will minimize medical errors. (PME)
Explaining the procedure	Ease the patient. (PBR)
Obtaining an inform consent	Respecting patients decision. (PS) (PBR)
Entering patient information (EKG unit)	To maintain the accuracy after the procedure. (PME)
Appropriate clothing	For proper electrode contact to the skin & to maintain patient privacy at the same time. (PS)
Standard precautions	Washing hands & wearing gloves helps in preventing cross infection. (SP)
Patient position	Standard patient position for recording an EKG (*supine*). (PS)
Electrode placement	Locating proper anatomical sites for limb and chest electrodes. (PME) (PS)
Skin preparation	To minimize skin impedance & get an artifact free EKG recording. (PME)
Application of electrode	For conduction of electrical activity of the heart. (PS)
Using alligator clips	To appropriately secure the alligator clips onto the electrodes. (PS)
Patient relaxation	• Inform the patient to avoid moving & talking during the procedure. (PS) • For standard recording have the patient maintain normal breathing pattern
Record	Print the EKG. (DOCU)
Check for calibration	Standard calibration and filter setting are used as required (PS)
Look for artifact	Look for any artifact (PS) if found: redo the procedure again
Disconnect alligator clips	On completion, disconnect the alligator clips from the electrodes and mount the cables appropriately. (PS)
Remove electrodes	Removal of electrode should be performed gently from the surface of the skin.(PS)
Remove gloves	Dispose the gloves. (SP)
Give patient privacy	Give the patient some time to dress. (PS)
Storing	Maintain the EKG recording in the patient file or in an appropriate location specified as per the facility guidelines. (DOCU)

PBR: Patients bill of rights   PME Prevent Medical Errors   PS: Procedural Standard   SP:Standard Precuations   Docu:Documentation

EQUIPMENT USE AND MAINTENANCE

Maintaining the EKG device

1. Any failure or defect in the machine should be reported.
2. Machine should be checked for cable damages and should be replaced immediately.
3. Check the machines for settings and outputs.
4. Check to see if the power socket is in working condition.
5. Clean the cables and machine using the manufacturer instructions and departmental policies.

INFECTION CONTROL IN EKG RECORDING
Chain of infection

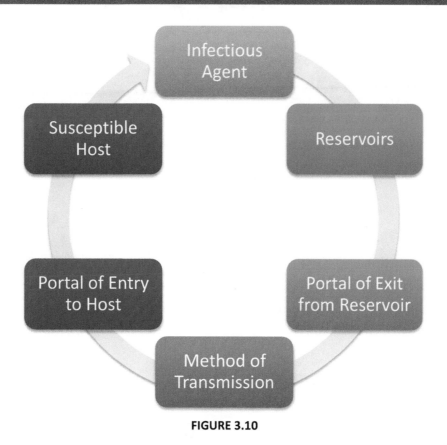

FIGURE 3.10

METHOD OF TRANSMISSION
An infectious agent may be transmitted from its reservoir to a susceptible host in different ways.

Direct Transmission

- Direct contact
- Droplet spread

Indirect Transmission

- Airborne
- Vehicle borne
- Vector borne (mechanical or biologic)

Steps in performing hand hygiene

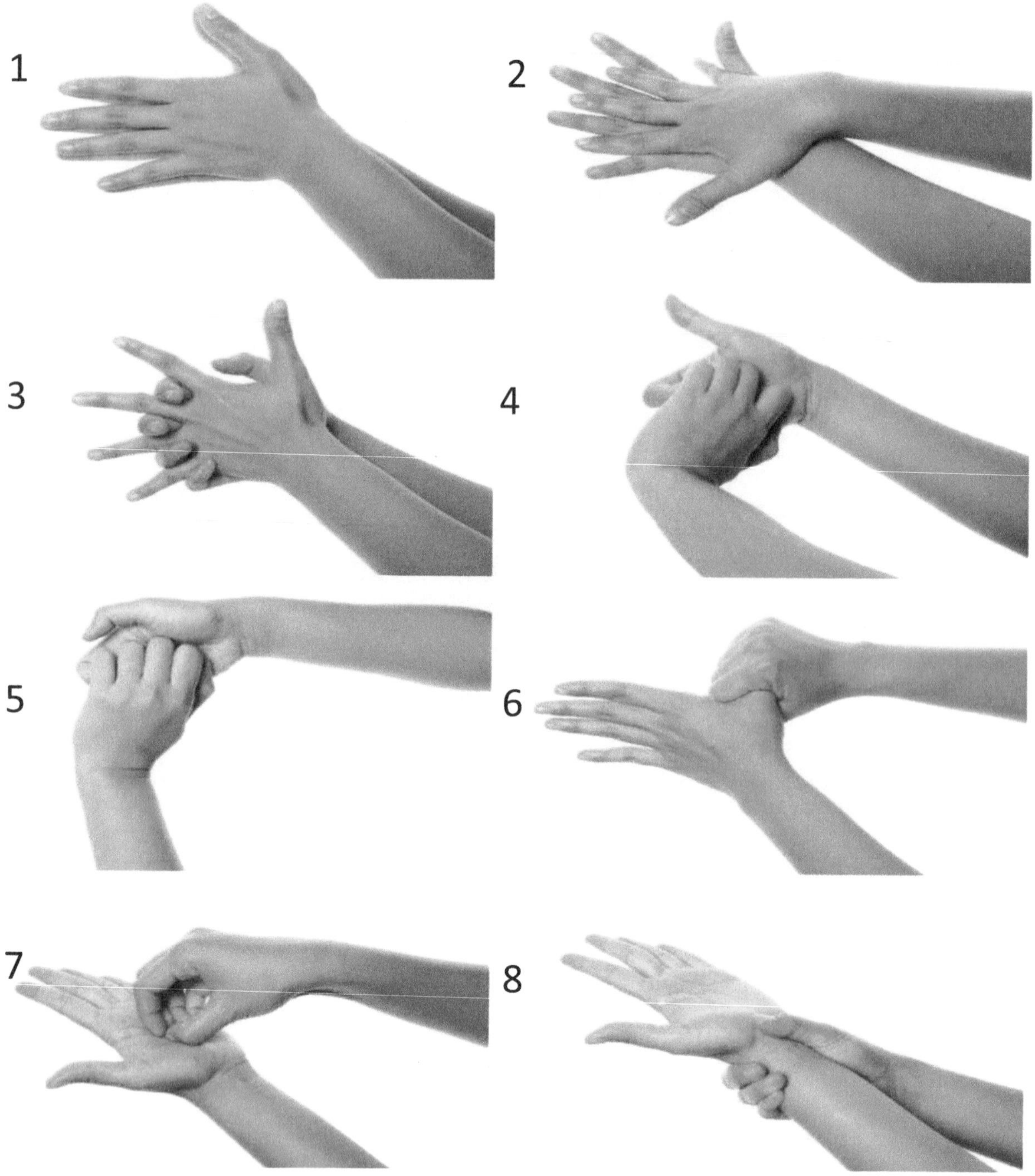

Hypo-allergic, antimicrobial soaps or alcohol based rubs can be used to perform the hand hygiene

FIGURE 3.11

IDENTIFYING EKG ARTIFACTS AND RECTIFYING THEM

Table 3.2 MUSCLE ARTIFACT

LOOK FOR	WHAT CAN BE DONE
If the patient is getting the EKG done for the first time they might be tensed.	Make sure that you explain the procedure, this may calm the patient and reduce anxiety. Respect the patient and cover them appropriately.
Some patients might clench the bed or the sheet on the bed during the procedure.	Inform the patient to relax during the procedure.
Check if the patient is able to follow your directions?	• The patient may have problems with concentration and may be tensed during the procedure. • Talking to the patient can help in gaining better concentration. • Check for assistance if required.
Check to see if the patient is moving	Some patients might feel cold due to the weather and start shivering, covering the patient with appropriate clothing (gown or other cloth) or perform the procedure in another room with suitable temperature
Neurological conditions	• Some neurological conditions might cause the patients to shiver. • Place the patients arm behind his or her back. • Place a pillow under the knee as this position may cause some relaxation. • Perform the procedure when the tremers are minimum or not present.*(parkinsonism)* • Use a filter setting if required.
Bed should be able to support the patient	• If the bed is too narrow, the patient will constantly try & balance his or her body on the bed in-order to be stable. • Make sure that the bed should have enough space so that the arms and feets are relaxed.

Table 3.3 MOVEMENT ARTIFACT

LOOK FOR	WHAT CAN BE DONE
Check to see if the patient is moving or not	Some patients may move the limbs while the procedure is being performed. If yes instruct the patient to lie still.
Check to see if the patient is talking or not	If yes, ask the patient to avoid talking during the

	procedure.
Check to see if the patient is chewing something	If yes explain the patient that movement during the EKG process may lead to performing the procedure again.
Cable tension	• Make sure that there is no tension in the cable to which the electrodes are applied as this may cause movement and pulling effect on the electrodes leading to detachment of electrodes from the skin surface completely or partially. • Cables should be detangled to avoid tension.
Cable suspended or hanging	Make sure that the cables are kept in a stationary position as their movement can also pull off the electrodes partially or completely displacing the electrodes from their standard locations.
Length of cables	Tall patients may need cables which are longer in length.
Patient age	• Pediatric patients should be kept in still position by distracting them with toys or with the most appropriate option available. • Ask the guardian or parents to hold the arms or legs gently to stop the movement.

Table 3.4 RESPIRATION ARTIFACT	
LOOK FOR	WHAT CAN BE DONE
Check to see if the patient is suffering from any respiratory condition which might have an effect on the procedure	Make sure to follow standard procedure to proceed. • If the patient is breathing too deep. • If the patient has difficulty breathing in supine position.
Check to see if the patient has discomfort breathing in supine position	Have the patient in semi-fowler position to minimize the discomfort of breathing.
Is the patient • Yawning • Coughing • Sneezing • Hiccups	Wait for yawning, hiccups, coughing or sneezing to subside.

Table 3.5 SKIN ARTIFACT

LOOK FOR	WHAT CAN BE DONE
Check to see if proper steps are followed	Standard steps should be followed for preparing the skin.
Hairy skin	• Follow standard procedure to remove the hair. • Use a hair clipper and cut the hair in the direction of the growth. • Cleanse the skin after removing the hair.
Oily skin	• Follow standard procedure to remove the oily remains on the surface of the skin. • Cleanse the area using alcohol pads or mild soap solution.
Diaphoresis	• Remove the sweat from the surface of the skin before the application of electrodes. • Set room temperature if possible.

Table 3.6 EKG EQUIPMENT ARTIFACT

LOOK FOR	WHAT CAN BE DONE
Check to see the expiration date of the electrodes	If expired use new electrodes.
Check to see the condition of the cables	If cables are damage or frayed replace with a new set.
Check to see the LCD display	If the EKG LCD display is not working follow the manufacturer instructions.
Check to see if the device is able to record the EKG	Sometimes the device may not function properly, reading the instruction manual provided by the manufacturer, may help in resolving the issue.
Check to see if the paper roll is moving while an EKG is being recorded	Incomplete closure of paper roll compartment may lead to the obstruction in the rolling movement of the paper roll.
Check to see if the paper roll has been installed correctly as per manufacturer instructions	Incorrect installation of the paper roll may lead to non-functioning of the paper roll while recording.
Check to see if other settings on the equipment are working satisfactorily	If not bring the EKG unit to its standard settings.
Check to see if the alligator clips are holding the electrodes	Partial clipping of the electrodes into the alligator clip may cause artifacts, make sure to completely clip the alligator clip to the tail of the electrode.

Table 3.7 INTERFERENCE ARTIFACT

LOOK FOR	WHAT CAN BE DONE
Are there any electronic devices in the nearby area causing an artifact	If yes, ask to see if your department has a specific guideline to deal with such situations if any.
Is the patient wearing an artificial pacemaker	If yes, perform the procedure as per standard protocol.
Is the patient wearing a hearing aid	If yes, the device can be switched off temporarily.

Table 3.8 ELECTRODE ARTIFACT

LOOK FOR	WHAT CAN BE DONE
Check the placement of the limb and chest electrodes. Check to see the progression of waveforms from V1 to V6.	If not, make sure that the electrodes are placed as per standard electrode placement.
Check to see if the alligator clips are properly secured to the electrodes	If not, make sure that the alligator clips are completely secured onto the electrodes.
Check to see if the electrodes are secured properly on the skin	If not, firmly press the electrodes against the skin to make sure that the electrodes are completely secured onto the skin surface. Pressure applied while trying to secure the electrodes should be light (should not be painful or cause any type of discomfort to the patient).

Table 3.9 MISSING ELECTRODE ARTIFACT

LOOK FOR	WHAT CAN BE DONE
LEAD I	Check to see if **Right Arm(RA)** & **Left Arm(LA)** electrodes are completely secured on to the surface of the skin and placed on the correct anatomical location.
LEAD II	Check to see if **Right Arm(RA)** & **Left Leg(LL)** electrodes are completely secured on to the surface of the skin and placed on the correct anatomical location.
LEAD III	Check to see if **Left Arm(LA)** & **Left Leg(LL)** electrodes are completely secured on to the surface of the skin and placed on the correct anatomical location.
LEAD aVR	Check to see if the **Right Arm(RA)** electrode is completely secured on to the surface of the skin and placed on the correct anatomical location.
LEAD aVL	Check to see if the **Left Arm(LA)** electrode is completely secured on to the surface of the skin and placed on the correct anatomical location.
LEAD aVF	Check to see if the **Left Leg(LL)** electrode is completely secured on to the surface of the skin

and placed on the correct anatomical location.

LEAD V1	Check to see if **V1 electrode** is completely secured on to the surface of the skin and placed on the correct anatomical location.
LEAD V2	Check to see if **V2 electrode** is completely secured on to the surface of the skin and placed on the correct anatomical location.
LEAD V3	Check to see if **V3 electrode** is completely secured on to the surface of the skin and placed on the correct anatomical location.
LEAD V4	Check to see if **V4 electrode** is completely secured on to the surface of the skin and placed on the correct anatomical location.
LEAD V5	Check to see if **V5 electrode** is completely secured on to the surface of the skin and placed on the correct anatomical location.
LEAD V6	Check to see if **V6 electrode** is completely secured on to the surface of the skin and placed on the correct anatomical location.

Table 3.10 12 LEAD EKG – HEART VIEW	
LOOK FOR	**VIEW OF HEART**
LEAD I	Lateral View
LEAD II	Inferior View
LEAD III	Inferior View
LEAD aVR	None
LEAD aVL	Lateral View
LEAD aVF	Inferior View
LEAD V1	Septum View
LEAD V2	Septum View
LEAD V3	Anterior View
LEAD V4	Anterior View
LEAD V5	Lateral View
LEAD V6	Lateral View

Table 3.11 15 LEAD EKG – HEART VIEW	
LOOK FOR	**VIEW OF HEART**
LEAD I	Lateral View
LEAD II	Inferior View
LEAD III	Inferior View
LEAD aVR	None
LEAD aVL	Lateral View
LEAD aVF	Inferior View
LEAD V1	Septum View
LEAD V2	Septum View
LEAD V3	Anterior View
LEAD V4	Anterior View
LEAD V5	Lateral View
LEAD V6	Lateral View
LEAD V4R	Right Ventricle View
LEAD V8	Posterior Wall of Left Ventricle
LEAD V9	Posterior Wall of Left Ventricle

LEGAL ISSUES IN HEALTHCARE

Assault: Threatening or causing bodily injury to another person, it may be a crime or a tort.

Battery: Touching a patient without his or her consent is termed as a battery, it can either be a civil or criminal offense.

Comparative negligence: Both parties are involved and the compensation depends on the contribution of the negligence, the jury decides the percentage of fault and the compensation has to be paid based on the percentage of fault.

Contributory negligence: Cases in which the plaintiffs own negligence lead to the injury.

Damages: The amount of money that is awarded by a court or the jury as a compensation for the tort.

Duty: Duty of care that the defendant owed the plaintiff. (An obligation owed by the defendant to provide care)

Dereliction: Breaching the duty of care that was owed to the plaintiff by the defendant.

Injury: Bodily harm to the plaintiff by the defendant.

Direct Cause: Injury sustained was due to direct action of the defendant.

Fraud: Intentionally hiding the truth for unlawful gains.

Health Insurance Portability and Accountability Act of 1996 (HIPAA): Title II of HIPAA (Administrative Simplification) consists of the privacy or security rule. The main purpose of these rules is to keep a patient's health information confidential and secure.

Informed Consent: is a procedure in which the permission is granted from the patient prior to the start of a healthcare procedure.

Expressed Consent: is a consent in which the permission is expressed by the person in written or spoken words prior to the start of a healthcare procedure.

Implied Consent: is a consent in which the permission is not expressed but rather inferred by the person's action, signs, facts or by inaction or silence.

Malpractice: A substandard delivery of care by the healthcare provider causing injury to the patient.

Negligence: Legal cause of action resulting from a failure to exercise the care that a reasonable person would exercise in like, same or similar circumstances.

Respondeat Superior: Employers are liable for the actions of an employee within the course and scope of their employment.

Defamation: In general is a written or oral statement which causes harm to the reputation of a person or third party.

Slander: A defamatory statement presented in an oral or spoken format.

Libel: A defamatory statement which is presented in a published or written format.

CHAPTER 4

EKG CLINICAL COMPETENCY

ELECTRODE PLACEMENT IN DIFFERENT REGIONS OF THE CHEST

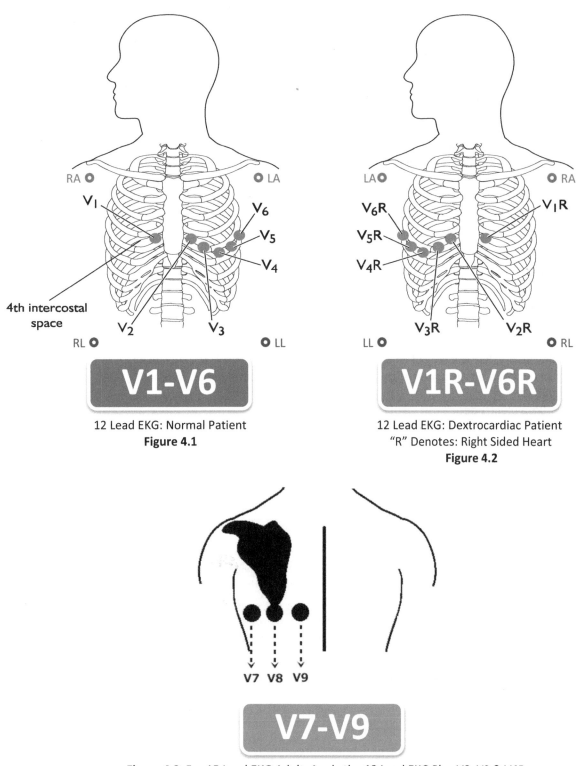

V1-V6

12 Lead EKG: Normal Patient
Figure 4.1

V1R-V6R

12 Lead EKG: Dextrocardiac Patient
"R" Denotes: Right Sided Heart
Figure 4.2

V7-V9

Figure 4.3 For 15 Lead EKG Adult: Apply the 12 Lead EKG Plus V8, V9 & V4R
For 15 Lead EKG Pediatric: Apply the 12 Lead EKG Plus V4R, V3R & V7

Important Note: The competency checklist has been designed only to provide general information. It is not intended to be comprehensive or provide any legal or medical advice. It is not recommended to replace any electrode placement recommended by the healthcare license professional. If it is an emergency **CALL 911**.

ELECTROCARDIOGRAPHY COMPETENCY CHECKLIST 12 LEAD EKG

Points to be awarded:	✓
1. Assemble and prepare equipment and supplies Check the speed on the EKG machine. It should be set to the standard reading of 25 mm/second, unless you are instructed otherwise. Make sure the unit is set to the full voltage. The unit will mark a standardization mark on the paper. Next, enter facility-required patient identification information. When performing the EKG, if part of a wave extends beyond the paper, reduce the normal standardization to half standardization. Note this adjustment on the EKG strip.	
2. Wash hands/don PPE (follow standard precautions)	
3. Greet the patient	
4. Identify yourself (name & designation)	
5. Identify patient (full name & date of birth)	
6. Explain procedure to the patient	
7. Position patient comfortably	
8. Prepare the skin for electrode placement a. If necessary, remove excess hair. Removing hair is usually not necessary, but excess hair will interfere with electrode adherence to the skin. Remove skin oil with the alcohol sponges, allow to dry. Rub the area of electrode placement briskly with a 4 x 4 gauze to abrade the area slightly. The area will appear slightly pink. This removes dead skin cells, promoting better contact	
9. Apply limb electrodes Position the limb electrodes. Connect the lead wires. For easy visual identification, each is color-coded and lettered.	
1) Right arm electrode labeled RA	
2) Right leg electrode labeled RL	
3) Left leg electrode labeled LL	
4) Left arm electrode labeled LA	
10. Apply precordial electrodes *(chest electrodes)* Apply electrodes to the chest. Avoid positioning the electrodes directly on bone. In the female, position the electrodes below the breast tissue. Palpate the clavicle (collarbone)and continue palpating downward to the fourth rib. Move down slightly to the space between the fourth and fifth ribs.	
• Position V1 electrode in the fourth intercostal space, to the right of the sternum.	
• Position V2 electrode directly opposite V1 at the left sternal border in 4th intercostal space	
• Next, position V4 electrode in the fifth intercostal space at the midclavicular line on left side	
• Position V3 electrode halfway between V2 and V4	
• Position V5 electrode and V6 laterally to V4	
• Position V5 electrode in the left anterior axillary line	
• Position V6 electrode in the left mid-axillary line	
11. Enter patient information into the EKG unit appropriately a. After applying the electrodes, enter information required by the facility into the EKG unit. Applying electrodes first allows the electrode gel to contact and penetrate the skin surface	

12. Correct for artifacts as appropriate (Check) ___ Muscle Artifact ___ 60 Cycle Interference ___Respiration ___Others if any (Specify)_____	
13. Ask the patient to lie still and breathe normally	
14. Select Print/Save on EKG machine to record the graph	
15. Once complete disconnect the electrodes from the patient while respecting the patients privacy	
16. Discard electrodes/contaminated items	
17. Wash hands / Thank the patient	
18. Document patient information and recorded graph	
19. Place/Mount EKG unit as appropriate (EKG Machine/Electrodes)	

ELECTROCARDIOGRAPHY COMPETENCY CHECKLIST 15 LEAD EKG: ADULT

Points to be awarded:	✓
1. Assemble and prepare equipment and supplies Check the speed on the EKG machine. It should be set to the standard reading of 25 mm/second, unless you are instructed otherwise. Make sure the unit is set to the full voltage. The unit will mark a standardization mark on the paper. Next, enter facility-required patient identification information. When performing the EKG, if part of a wave extends beyond the paper, reduce the normal standardization to half standardization. Note this adjustment on the EKG strip.	
2. Wash hands/don PPE (follow standard precautions)	
3. Greet the patient	
4. Identify yourself (name & designation)	
5. Identify patient (full name & date of birth)	
6. Explain procedure to the patient	
7. Position patient comfortably	
8. Prepare the skin for electrode placement If necessary, remove excess hair. Removing hair is usually not necessary, but excess hair will interfere with electrode adherence to the skin. Remove skin oil with the alcohol sponges, allow to dry. Rub the area of electrode placement briskly with a 4 x 4 gauze to abrade the area slightly. The area will appear slightly pink. This removes dead skin cells, promoting better contact	
9. Apply limb electrodes Position the limb electrodes. Connect the lead wires. For easy visual identification, each is color-coded and lettered.	
a. Right arm electrode labeled RA	
b. Right leg electrode labeled RL	
c. Left leg electrode labeled LL	
d. Left arm electrode labeled LA	
10. Apply precordial electrodes (chest electrodes) Apply electrodes to the chest. Avoid positioning the electrodes directly on bone. In the female, position the electrodes below the breast tissue. Palpate the clavicle (collarbone)and continue palpating downward to the fourth rib. Move down slightly to the space between the fourth and fifth ribs.	
• Position V1 electrode in the fourth intercostal space, to the right of the sternum.	

• Position V2 electrode directly opposite V1 at the left sternal border in 4th intercostal space	
• Next, position V4 electrode in the fifth intercostal space at the midclavicular line on left side	
• Position V3 electrode halfway between V2 and V4	
• Position V5 electrode and V6 laterally to V4	
• Position V5 electrode in the left anterior axillary line	
• Position V6 electrode in the left mid-axillary line	
• V4R position in the 5th intercostal space in the right anterior mid-clavicular line	
• V8 position in line laterally to V6 on 5th intercostal space, in the left mid-scapular line	
• V9 position laterally to V8, between V8 and spinal column at posterior 5th intercostal space	
11. Enter patient information into the EKG unit appropriately a. After applying the electrodes, enter information required by the facility into the EKG unit. Applying electrodes first allows the electrode gel to contact and penetrate the skin surface	
12. Correct for artifacts as appropriate (Check) ___ Muscle Artifact ___ 60 Cycle Interference ___Respiration ___Others if any (Specify)_____	
13. Ask the patient to lie still and breathe normally	
14. Select Print/Save on EKG machine to record the graph	
15. Once complete disconnect the electrodes from the patient while respecting the patients privacy	
16. Discard electrodes/contaminated items	
17. Wash hands / Thank the patient	
18. Document patient information and recorded graph	
19. Place/Mount EKG unit as appropriate (EKG Machine/Electrodes)	

ELECTROCARDIOGRAPHY COMPETENCY CHECKLIST 15 LEAD EKG: PEDIATRIC

Points to be awarded:	✓
1. Assemble and prepare equipment and supplies Check the speed on the EKG machine. It should be set to the standard reading of 25 mm/second, unless you are instructed otherwise. Make sure the unit is set to the full voltage. The unit will mark a standardization mark on the paper. Next, enter facility-required patient identification information. When performing the EKG, if part of a wave extends beyond the paper, reduce the normal standardization to half standardization. Note this adjustment on the EKG strip.	
2. Wash hands/don PPE (follow standard precautions)	
3. Greet the patient	
4. Identify yourself (name & designation)	
5. Identify patient (full name & date of birth)	
6. Explain procedure to the patient	
7. Position patient comfortably	
8. Prepare the skin for electrode placement If necessary, remove excess hair. Removing hair is usually not necessary, but excess hair will interfere with electrode adherence to the skin. Remove skin oil with the alcohol sponges, allow to dry. Rub the area of electrode placement briskly with a 4 x 4 gauze to abrade the area slightly. The area will appear slightly pink. This removes dead skin cells, promoting better contact	

9. Apply limb electrodes Position the limb electrodes. Connect the lead wires. For easy visual identification, each is color-coded and lettered.	
a. Right arm electrode labeled RA	
b. Right leg electrode labeled RL	
c. Left leg electrode labeled LL	
d. Left arm electrode labeled LA	
10. Apply precordial electrodes *(chest electrodes)* Apply electrodes to the chest. Avoid positioning the electrodes directly on bone. In the female, position the electrodes below the breast tissue. Palpate the clavicle (collarbone)and continue palpating downward to the fourth rib. Move down slightly to the space between the fourth and fifth ribs.	
• Position V1 electrode in the fourth intercostal space, to the right of the sternum.	
• Position V2 electrode directly opposite V1 at the left sternal border in 4th intercostal space	
• Next, position V4 electrode in the fifth intercostal space at the midclavicular line on left side	
• Position V3 electrode halfway between V2 and V4	
• Position V5 electrode and V6 laterally to V4	
• Position V5 electrode in the left anterior axillary line	
• Position V6 electrode in the left mid-axillary line	
• V4R position in the 5th intercostal space in the right anterior midclavicular line	
• V3R position between V1 and V4R	
• V7 position on posterior axillary line in line with V5 & V6	
11. Enter patient information into the EKG unit appropriately a. After applying the electrodes, enter information required by the facility into the EKG unit. Applying electrodes first allows the electrode gel to contact and penetrate the skin surface	
12. Correct for artifacts as appropriate (Check) ___ Muscle Artifact ___ 60 Cycle Interference ___Respiration ___Others if any (Specify)_____	
13. Ask the patient to lie still and breathe normally	
14. Select Print/Save on EKG machine to record the graph	
15. Once complete disconnect the electrodes from the patient while respecting the patients privacy	
16. Discard electrodes/contaminated items	
17. Wash hands / Thank the patient	
18. Document patient information and recorded graph	
19. Place/Mount EKG unit as appropriate (EKG Machine/Electrodes)	

HOLTERS MONITORING: 5 LEAD COMPETENCY CHECKLIST

Points to be awarded:	✓
1. Assemble and prepare equipment & supplies	
2. Holter monitor preparation 　a. Installing Battery 　b. Installing Recorder Memory (Flash Card or Cassette)	
3. Greet the patient	
4. Identify yourself (name & designation)	
5. Identify patient (full name & date of birth)	
6. Explain procedure to the patient & guidelines of Holters Monitoring	
7. Position patient comfortably and have the patient expose the chest area	
8. Prepare the skin for electrode placement If necessary, remove excess hair. Removing hair is usually not necessary, but excess hair will interfere with electrode adherence to the skin. Remove skin oil with the alcohol sponges, allow to dry. Rub the area of electrode placement briskly with a 4 x 4 gauze to abrade the area slightly. The area will appear slightly pink. This removes dead skin cells, promoting better contact	
9. Apply electrodes & explain the patient about why the electrodes should always be in contact for the time of recording (Check next page for electrode placements)	
10. Attach lead wires to electrodes.	
11. Form a loop in each lead wire.	
12. Attach loop to the patient with a tape	
13. Placed tape over each electrode	
14. Connect lead wires to patient cable	
15. Check the recorder using the test cable connected to an ECG machine and running a short baseline recording to see if the device is in a working condition	
16. Next Instruct the patient to dress & how to properly position cable	
17. Insert recording unit in a case and then strapped it to the patients cloth	
18. Next plug electrode cables into the recorder unit & turn on the recording unit	
19. Record the start time of the unit	
20. Instruct the patient on how to complete the dairy	
21. Inform the patient when to return for removing the recording unit	
22. Wash hands / Thank the patient	
23. Document patient information	

OPTION 1

HOLTER MONITORING 3 CHANNEL (5 LEAD) ELECTRODE PLACEMENT

#	Channel	Color	Placement
1	3-	White	Below the clavicle, next to the right clavicle border
2	1-, 2-	Red	Top of the sternum, over the manubrium
3	2+, 3+	Black	Left midclavicular line,8th rib
4	1+	Brown	Left anterior axillary line over the 5th or 6th rib (as per physicians order)
5	Ground	Green	Right midclavicular line,8th rib

```
BROWN   –   RED     +    = CHANNEL 1
BLACK   –   RED     +    = CHANNEL 2
BLACK   –   WHITE   +    = CHANNEL 3
```

OPTION 2

HOLTER MONITORING 3 CHANNEL (5 LEAD) ELECTRODE PLACEMENT

#	Channel	Color	Placement
1	3-	White	Right side below the V1 position, at the bottom of the rib cage
2	1-, 2-	Red	Center on the Manubrium, the top of the sternum
3	2+, 3+	Black	Left side at the V5 position, on the 8th rib
4	1+	Brown	Left side at the V3 position, on the 8th rib
5	Ground	Green	Right side opposite V5 position, on the lower rib cage.

```
RED     –   BROWN +    = CHANNEL 1
RED     –   BLACK +    = CHANNEL 2
WHITE   –   BLACK +    = CHANNEL 3
```

PLACEMENT FOR HOLTERS MONITORING MAY CHANGES AS PER THE PHYSICIANS OR PROVIDERS REQUEST

TELEMETRY ELECTRODE PLACEMENTS

5 LEAD TELEMETRY	
RA	Right Arm
LA	Left Arm
RL	Right Leg
LL	Left Leg
V1	4th intercostal space on right of sternum

Nursing Homes

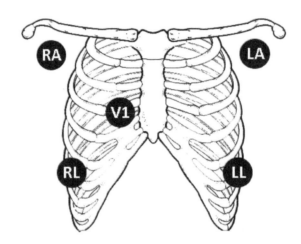

FIGURE 4.4

3 LEAD TELEMETRY	
RA	Right Arm
LA	Left Arm
LL	Left Leg

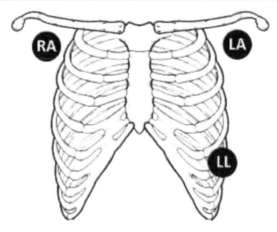

FIGURE 4.5

EXERCISE STRESS TEST

Electrode	Placement
V1	Position V1 electrode in the fourth intercostal space, to the right of the sternum.
V2	Position V2 electrode directly opposite V1 at the left sternal border in 4th intercostal space
V3	Position V3 electrode halfway between V2 and V4
V4	Next, position V4 electrode in the fifth intercostal space at the midclavicular line on left side
V5	Position V5 electrode in the left anterior axillary line, in line with V4
V6	Position V6 electrode in the left mid-axillary line
RA	Below the right clavicle
LA	Below the left clavicle
RL	On the right lower edges of rib cage or same level at umbilicus at midclavicular line
LL	On the left lower edges of rib cage or same level at umbilicus at midclavicular line

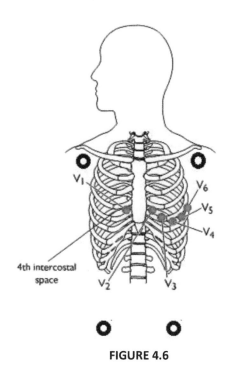

FIGURE 4.6

Chapter 4: EKG CLINICAL COMPETENCY

HOW TO PERFORM AN EXERCISE STRESS TEST

What is monitored during the exercise stress test?

Pulse Rate

Respiratory Rate

Blood Pressure

Electrocardiogram

Rate of Perceived Exertion

Few Indications to Exercise Stress Testing

Irregular heart beat

Chest pain or angina

Dyspnea

Diagnosis of coronary heart disease

Post myocardial infarction for activity prescription and prognostic assessment

Determination of exercise capacity of patients with valvular heart disease

Few Contraindications to Exercise Stress Testing

Acute myocardial infarction or unstable angina

Acute cardiac inflammation

Pericarditis

Endocarditis

Myocarditis

Severe congestive heart failure

Uncontrolled sustained ventricular arrhythmias

Severe hypertension

Pulmonary embolism

Deep venous thrombosis

Poor candidate for exercise

Extremely obese

Severe mental or physical disabilities

Electrolyte abnormalities

How is the test performed?

— Perform the steps 1-10 of the procedure mentioned in the 12 lead EKG competency checklists, for electrode placement refer to (figure 4.6)

— A blood pressure cuff is placed on the patients arm.

— A pulse oximetry may be attached to the finger of the patient to record the oxygen saturation during the procedure.

— A baseline EKG, blood pressure & pulse are recorded before asking the patient to start the graded exercise.

— The patient will then be asked to perform graded exercise by either walking on a treadmill or on a stationary bike.*(Treadmill, Cycle Ergometer or Steps, equipments used may vary depending on the patient's condition to use the equipments and also on availability of the equipments).*

— Every 3 minutes the patient's EKG and Non-EKG parameters like blood pressure, pulse, respiratory rate are recorded with any symptoms if the patient experiences during the graded exercise.

The exercise stress test can be performed at a

- **Sub-maximal level by following the**

    o   Sub-maximal exercise testing protocol

- **Maximal level by following the**

    o   Maximal exercise testing protocol

Indications for termination of exercise stress test

- Moderate to severe chest pain
- Fatigue or difficulty breathing
- Fainting or dizziness
- Cyanosis
- On the request of the patient
- ST segment depression (Excessive)
- Excessive hypertension
- Drop in the systolic blood pressure with increase in activity
- Leg cramps or claudication

Post exercise stress testing recordings can be taken in sitting position or recumbent position.

National Certification Career Association

EKG Practical – Log Sheet

Student's Name: _____

Facility Name: _____

Supervisor's Name: _____

1. EKG TYPE	Successful	Unsuccessful	Supervisor Initials Date: / /
2. EKG TYPE	Successful	Unsuccessful	Supervisor Initials Date: / /
3. EKG TYPE	Successful	Unsuccessful	Supervisor Initials Date: / /
4. EKG TYPE	Successful	Unsuccessful	Supervisor Initials Date: / /
5. EKG TYPE	Successful	Unsuccessful	Supervisor Initials Date: / /
6. EKG TYPE	Successful	Unsuccessful	Supervisor Initials Date: / /
7. EKG TYPE	Successful	Unsuccessful	Supervisor Initials Date: / /
8. EKG TYPE	Successful	Unsuccessful	Supervisor Initials Date: / /
9. EKG TYPE	Successful	Unsuccessful	Supervisor Initials Date: / /
10. EKG TYPE	Successful	Unsuccessful	Supervisor Initials Date: / /

Total Successful EKG _____ / Page

SHEET NUMBER (CIRCLE):   1   2   3   4

Check sign in appropriate boxes	✓

MAKE COPIES AS NEEDED

Printed by permission from National Certification Career Association NCCA www.nccanow.com

Chapter 4: EKG CLINICAL COMPETENCY

CHAPTER 5

EKG PRACTICE EXAM

EKG   Exam   Section:

Practice Test

Questions: 100

1. The human heart consists of_____4_____ Valves
   A) 1
   B) 2
   C) 3
   D) 4

2. Sac surrounding the heart is_____
   A) Pericardium
   B) Myocardium
   C) Epicardium
   D) Endocardium

3. The innermost layer of the heart is _____
   A) Pericardium
   B) Endocardium
   C) Myocardium
   D) Epicardium

4. The outermost layer of the heart _____
   A) Pericardium
   B) Myocardium
   C) Epicardium
   D) Endocardium

5. The middle layer of the heart is _____
   A) Pericardium
   B) Myocardium
   C) Endocardium
   D) Epicardium

6. The muscular layer of the heart is _____
   A) Pericardium
   B) Endocardium
   C) Myocardium
   D) Epicardium

7. Which of the following are Bipolar Leads:
   A) Lead I, II, III
   B) Lead I, II, VI
   C) Lead III, IV, V
   D) Lead IV, V, VI

8. Which of the following are Unipolar Leads:
   A) aVR, aVL and aVF
   B) lead I, II, and III
   C) lead I and II
   D) lead II and III

Chapter 5: EKG CERTIFICATION EXAM REVIEW

9. Which of the following are Precordial Leads?
   A) V1-V6
   B) V2-V6
   C) V3-V6
   D) None of the above

10. Placement of V_1 electrode in a 12 Lead EKG would be:
   A) 4th intercostal space to left of the sternum
   B) 4th intercostal space to right of the sternum
   C) 4th intercostal space left midclavicular line
   D) None of the above

11. Placement of V_2 electrode in a 12 Lead EKG would be:
   A) 4th intercostal space to the left of the sternum
   B) 4th intercostal space to the right of the sternum
   C) 5th intercostal space to the right of the sternum
   D) Between V1 and V3

12. Placement of V_3 electrode in a 12 Lead EKG would be:
   A) 4th intercostal space to the right of the sternum
   B) 5th intercostal space to the left the sternum
   C) Between V2 and V4
   D) Between V1 and V2

13. P wave morphology can be best described by:
   A) The first wave seen
   B) The wave following the QRS complex
   C) The wave following the T wave
   D) None of the above

14. T wave morphology can be best described by:
   A) The first wave seen
   B) The rounded upright wave following the QRS
   C) The small rounded, upright following the QRS
   D) None of the above

15. PR interval morphology can be best described by:
   A) Distance between beginning of P wave and beginning of QRS
   B) Distance beginning of P wave and T wave
   C) Distance between S wave and T wave
   D) None of the above

16. QT interval morphology can be best described by:
   A) Distance between Q wave and P wave
   B) Measured from beginning of QRS to end of T wave √
   C) Measured from beginning of P to end of R wave
   D) Measured from beginning of S to end of Q wave

17. U wave morphology can be best described by:
  A) Small rounded, upright wave following T wave
  B) Small rounded, upright wave following S wave
  C) Small rounded, upright wave following P wave
  D) None of the above

18. Placement of V_4 electrode in a 12 Lead EKG would be:
  A) Midway between V2 and V4
  B) 5th intercostal space at the left midclavicular line
  C) 5th intercostal space at the right midclavicular line
  D) None of the above

19. Placement of V_5 electrode in a 12 Lead EKG would be:
  A) 5th intercostal space at the left mid-clavicular line
  B) 5th intercostal space at the left mid-axillary line
  C) 5th intercostal space at the left anterior axillary line
  D) 5th intercostal space at the left of the sternum

20. Placement of V_6 electrode in a 12 Lead EKG would be:
  A) 5th intercostal space at the left mid-axillary line
  B) 5th intercostal space at the right of the sternum
  C) 5th intercostal space at the left of the sternum
  D) 5th intercostal space at the left mid-clavicular line

21. QRS complex morphology can be best described by: _following_
  A) Deflections of 3 waves followed by the P wave
  B) Distance between S wave and T wave
  C) Distance between P wave and U wave
  D) Distance between Q wave and T wave

22. ST segment morphology can be best described by:
  A) Distance between S wave and beginning of the T wave
  B) Distance between P wave and T wave
  C) Distance between P wave and U wave
  D) None of the above

23. What is a cardiac cycle?
  A) Sequence of event in 1 heartbeat. Blood is pumped through the entire cardiovascular system.
  B) Sequence of event in 1 heartbeat. Blood is ejected from either ventricle in single contraction
  C) Amount of blood pumped through the cardiovascular system in one minute
  D) None of the above

24. A Systole can be identified as the:
  A) Contraction phase
  B) Relaxation phase
  C) Sequence of event in one heartbeat
  D) None of the above

Chapter 5: EKG CERTIFICATION EXAM REVIEW

25. Stroke volume can be described as:
- A) Sequence of event in 1 heartbeat
- B) Amount of blood pumped through the cardiovascular system per minute
- C) Amount of blood ejected from either ventricle in a single contraction
- D) None of the above

26. A Diastole can be identified as the:
- A) Contraction phase
- B) Relaxation phase
- C) Sequence of event in 1 heartbeat
- D) None of the above

27. Which of the following option best describe the Cardiac Output:
- A) Amount of blood pumped through the cardiovascular system in 1 minute
- B) Amount of blood ejected from an atrium in a single contraction
- C) Amount of blood ejected from either ventricle in a single contraction
- D) None of the above

28. Which of the following is a property of a cardiac cell?
- A) Automaticity
- B) Excitability
- C) Conductivity
- D) All of the above

29. Heart is located in the:
- A) Mediastinum
- B) Stomach
- C) Abdomen
- D) None of the above

30. Ventricle are the:
- A) Lower chambers of the heart
- B) Upper chamber of the heart
- C) Layer of the heart
- D) Right sided chambers of the heart

31. Which of the following is not a commonly seen wave on an EKG tracing?
- A) P wave
- B) Q wave
- C) T wave
- D) U wave

32. The ability of the heart to create its own electrical impulse would be termed:
- A) Conductivity
- B) Contractility
- C) Automaticity
- D) Excitability

33. Which of the following option best describe de-oxygenated blood?
   A) Blood having oxygen
   B) Blood having no oxygen
   C) Lack of blood
   D) None of the above

34. Which of the following option best describe oxygenated blood?
   A) Blood having oxygen
   B) Blood having non oxygen
   C) Lack of blood
   D) None of the above

35. Range for normal heartbeat would be between:
   A) 50 to 120
   B) 40 to 100
   C) 50 to 100
   D) 60 to 100

36. Bradycardia can be described as:
   A) Slow heart rate
   B) Fast heart rate
   C) No heart rate
   D) Regular heart rate

37. Tachycardia can be described as:
   A) Slow heart rate
   B) Fast heart rate
   C) No heart rate
   D) Regular heart rate

38. Which of the following is the most important step in performing an EKG?
   A) Identify yourself
   B) Identify the patient
   C) Ask if the patient has ever had the procedure before and explain the procedure
   D) All of the above

39. Which of the following is the correct statement?
   A) 1 big square equal 5 small squares
   B) 1 small square equal 5 big squares
   C) 1 big square equal 6 small squares
   D) 1 big square equal 4 small squares

changed

40. Which of the following is the correct statement?
   A) 1 big square = 0.02 sec
   B) 1 small square = 0.20 sec
   C) 1 small square = 0.04 sec
   D) None of the above

41. A 0.20 sec on an EKG tracing is equal to:
   A) 1 big square
   B) 1 small squares
   C) 2 big squares
   D) 5 big square

42. Which of the following describes **Heart Rate**?
   A) The number of time the heart beats per minute
   B) The contraction of the heart
   C) The relaxation of the heart
   D) The number of time the heart beat a day

43. Most common way for assessing a regular rhythm on a EKG tracing would be to count:
   A) The number of large boxes between 2 T waves
   B) The number of large boxes between 2 P waves
   C) The number of large boxes between 2 R waves
   D) None of the above

44. Which method should be used to calculate heart rate when using large boxes as reference in a 6sec EKG tracing:
   A) 300 ÷ number of boxes
   B) 3000 ÷ number of boxes
   C) 150 ÷ number of boxes
   D) 1500 ÷ number of boxes

45. Which method should be used to calculate heart rate when using small boxes as reference in a 6sec EKG tracing:
   A) 300 ÷ number of boxes
   B) 3000 ÷ number of boxes
   C) 150 ÷ number of boxes
   D) 1500 ÷ number of boxes

46. If the distance between 2 "R" waves is 15 small boxes, the heart rate would be interpreted as :
   A) 50 bpm
   B) 100 bpm
   C) 150 bpm
   D) 125 bpm

47. If the distance between 2 "R" waves is 10 small boxes, the heart rate would be interpreted as:
   A) 150 bpm
   B) 100 bpm
   C) 125 bpm
   D) 75 bpm

48. If the distance between 2 "R" waves is 5 small boxes, the heart rate would be interpreted as:
   A) 100 bpm
   B) 200 bpm
   C) 250 bpm
   D) 300 bpm

Chapter 5: EKG CERTIFICATION EXAM REVIEW

49. If the distance between 2 "R" waves is 5 large boxes, the heart rate would be interpreted as:
- A) 40 bpm
- B) 50 bpm
- C) 60 bpm
- D) 70 bpm

50. If the distance between 2 "R" waves is 10 large boxes, the heart rate would be interpreted as:
- A) 30 bpm
- B) 40 bpm
- C) 50 bpm
- D) 60 bpm

51. If the distance between 2 "R" waves is 15 large boxes, the heart rate would be interpreted as:
- A) 20 bpm
- B) 30 bpm
- C) 40 bpm
- D) 50 bpm

52. Which of the following can be interpreted by EKG:
- A) Rate
- B) Regularity
- C) P wave
- D) All of the above

53. Sinus bradycardia would most likely have a heart rate of:
- A) >60 bpm
- B) <60 bpm
- C) > 100 bpm
- D) < 100 bpm

54. Sinus tachycardia would most likely have a heart rate of:
- A) > 60 bpm
- B) < 60 bpm
- C) > 100 bpm
- D) < 100 bpm

55. Most common type of EKG application used in a physician office setting would be:
- A) 3 leads
- B) 5 leads
- C) 12 leads
- D) 15 leads

56. The location of Sino-Atrial is:
- A) Upper portion of the right atrium
- B) Upper portion of the right ventricle
- C) Upper portion of the left atrium
- D) Lower portion of the right atrium

Chapter 5: EKG CERTIFICATION EXAM REVIEW

57. The location of Internodal pathway is:
   A) Between SA and AV node
   B) In lower portion of the left ventricle
   C) In lower portion of the left atrium
   D) None of the above

58. Which of the following statements below describe the function of internodal pathway:
   A) To create a slight delay before impulses reach ventricles
   B) Conduct impulse that lead to the left ventricle
   C) Direct electrical impulses between SA and AV nodes
   D) None of the above

59. Bundle of His is located:
   A) Below AV node
   B) Above AV node
   C) Below SA node
   D) Above SA node

60. The function of the left bundle branch is to:
   A) Conduct impulses to the left ventricle
   B) Conduct impulses to the right ventricle
   C) Transmit impulses to bundle branches
   D) All of the above

61. Which of the following describes the function of Bundle of His:
   A) Conduct impulses to the left ventricle
   B) Conduct impulses to the right ventricle
   C) Transmit impulse to bundle branches
   D) None of the above

62. The location of Purkinje system:
   A) Terminals of bundle branches
   B) The left ventricle
   C) Left atrium
   D) None of the above

63. The function of the right bundle branch is to:
   A) Conduct impulse to the left ventricle
   B) Conduct impulse to the left atrium
   C) Conduct impulse to the right atrium
   D) Conduct impulse to the right ventricle

64. Lead V_1-V_6 are which of the following leads:
   A) Bipolar lead
   B) Tripolar lead
   C) Unipolar lead
   D) None of the above

65. Which of the following are considered standard leads in a 12 lead EKG Tracing:
   A) aVR, aVL, aVF
   B) lead I,II,III
   C) V1-V6
   D) All of the above

66. Which of the following are considered augmented leads in a 12 lead EKG Tracing:
   A) aVR, aVL, aVF
   B) lead I, II, III
   C) V1-V6
   D) All of the above

67. Which of the following would be termed as an ability of the heart to respond to an electrical stimulus?
   A) Automaticity
   B) Excitability
   C) Conductivity
   D) Contractility

68. The ability of the heart to generate electrical impulse independently, without involving the nervous system is called:
   A) Automaticity
   B) Excitability
   C) Conductivity
   D) Contractility

69. The ability of the heart to pass or propagate electrical impulses from one cell to another cell is termed as:
   A) Automaticity
   B) Excitability
   C) Conductivity
   D) Contractility

70. The ability of the heart to shorten in response to an electrical stimulation would be termed:
   A) Automaticity
   B) Excitability
   C) Conductivity
   D) Contractility

71. On a 12 lead EKG Tracing a normal PR interval is:
   A) 0.10-0.20 sec
   B) 0.12-0.20 sec
   C) 0.10-0.02 sec
   D) 0.01-0.20 sec

72. On a 12 lead EKG Tracing a normal QRS interval varies between:
   A) 0.5 - 0.10 sec
   B) 0.6 - 0.10 sec
   C) 0.06 - 0.10 sec
   D) 0.5 - 0.010 sec

73. Prior to applying electrodes on the patient skin, which is the most appropriate step taken by the EKG technician for better skin contact?
   A) Wipe the skin with alcohol pad and then apply electrodes
   B) Briskly scrub the skin with rough paper and wipe it with alcohol pad
   C) Wash the skin with soap
   D) Wash the skin with luke warm saline water

74. Which of the following is a negative wave?
   A) P wave
   B) T wave
   C) U wave
   D) Q wave

75. Prior to performing an EKG you should:
   A) Check the patient name and ID number
   B) Verified the patient date of birth
   C) Check the medical record
   D) All of the above

76. Which of the following chamber of the heart receives blood from the superior and inferior vena cava?
   A) Left atrium
   B) Left ventricle
   C) Right ventricle
   D) Right atrium

77. Which of the following chamber pumps the blood through the aortic valve?
   A) Left ventricle
   B) Right ventricle
   C) Left atrium
   D) Right atrium

78. Which of the following chamber pumps the blood through the mitral (bicuspid) valve?
   A) Left ventricle
   B) Left atrium
   C) Right atrium
   D) Right ventricle

79. Which of the following chamber pumps the blood through the tricuspid valve?
   A) Right atrium
   B) Left atrium
   C) Right ventricle
   D) Left ventricle

80. Deoxygenated blood is received by the right atrium through the:
   A) Superior vena cava
   B) Inferior vena cava
   C) Aorta
   D) Superior and inferior vena cava

81. The valve located between the left atrium and the left ventricle is:
   A) Mitral (bicuspid) valve
   B) Aortic valve
   C) Tricuspid valve
   D) Pulmonary valve

82. The valve located between the right atrium and the right ventricle is:
   A) Mitral (bicuspid) valve
   B) Aortic valve
   C) Tricuspid valve
   D) Pulmonary valve

83. The single most important way to stop the spread of infection is:
   A) Standard precaution
   B) Isolation procedure
   C) Hand hygiene
   D) PPE

84. The valve located between the left ventricle and the aorta:
   A) Mitral valve
   B) Aortic valve
   C) Tricuspid valve
   D) Pulmonary valve

85. The valve located between the right ventricle and the pulmonary artery?
   A) Mitral valve
   B) Aortic valve
   C) Tricuspid valve
   D) Pulmonary valve

86. The placement of the $V4_R$ electrode in a 15 lead EKG would be:
   A) 5th intercostal space in right anterior midclavicular line
   B) 5th intercostal space in left anterior midaxillary line
   C) 4th intercostal space in right anterior midaxillary line
   D) None of the above

87. The placement of the V_8 electrode in a 15 lead EKG would be:
   A) Anterior 5th intercostal space in left mid-scapular line
   B) Posterior 5th intercostal space in left mid-scapular line
   C) Posterior 5th intercostal space in left mid-clavicular line
   D) None of the above

88. The placement of the V_9 electrode in a 15 lead EKG would be:
   A) Anterior 5th intercostal space in left mid-clavicular line
   B) Directly between V8 and spinal column at posterior 5th intercostal space
   C) Directly between V6 and V9
   D) None of the above

Chapter 5: EKG CERTIFICATION EXAM REVIEW

89. The duration of a QRS complex in a Bundle Branch Block is:
   A) >0.10 sec
   B) <0.10 sec
   C) >0.20 sec
   D) <0.20 sec

90. Inferior vena cava receives blood from the:
   A) Lower part of the body
   B) Upper part of the body
   C) A and B
   D) None of the above

91. Superior vena cava receives blood from the:
   A) Lower part of the body
   B) Upper part of the body
   C) A and B
   D) None of the above

92. The prefix brady means:
   A) Slow
   B) Fast
   C) Normal
   D) None of the above

93. Amount of blood ejected from either ventricle in a single contraction _____
   A) The systole
   B) The cardiac cycle
   C) The stroke volume
   D) The cardiac output

94. Which of the following PACEMAKER generates an impulse of 40-60 bpm?
   A) The Atria
   B) The Purkinje fibers
   C) The SA node
   D) The AV node

95. The Frank-Starling law of the heart states that the:
   A) Degree of cardiac muscle stretched can increase the force of ejected blood
   B) Degree of cardiac muscle relaxed can decrease the force of ejected blood
   C) Degree of cardiac muscle stretched can decrease the force of ejected blood
   D) Degree of cardiac muscle relaxed can increase the force of ejected blood

96. The correct way to calculate the cardiac output (CO) is:
   A) CO= Stroke Volume x Heart Rate
   B) CO= Maximum Heart x Stroke Volume
   C) CO= Blood Pressure x Stroke Volume
   D) CO= Stroke volume x Respiratory Rate

Chapter 5: EKG CERTIFICATION EXAM REVIEW

97. To find a person's maximum heart rate or HR$_{MAX}$ the persons age must be subtracted by:
   A) 100-Age
   B) 220-Age
   C) 120-Age
   D) 200-Age

98. U wave represents:
   A) Represents repolarization of Purkinje fibers
   B) Represents depolarization of Purkinje fibers
   C) Represents repolarization of Sino-Atrial node
   D) Represents depolarization of Sino-Atrial node

99. ST segment:
   A) Measures time between atrial depolarization and beginning of ventricular repolarization
   B) Measures time between atrial depolarization and beginning of another atrial depolarization
   C) Measures time between ventricular depolarization and beginning of repolarization
   D) Measures time between ventricular repolarization and beginning of atrial depolarization

100. Which of the following best describes an EKG:
   A) Is the study of the heart
   B) Is a series of waves and deflections recording the heart's electrical activity from a certain view
   C) Is a disorder of the heart
   D) Is the study of electricity

Chapter 5: EKG CERTIFICATION EXAM REVIEW

ANSWER KEY

1.	D		51.	A
2.	A		52.	D
3.	B		53.	B
4.	C		54.	C
5.	B		55.	C
6.	C		56.	A
7.	A		57.	A
8.	A		58.	C
9.	A		59.	A
10.	B		60.	A
11.	A		61.	C
12.	C		62.	A
13.	A		63.	D
14.	B		64.	C
15.	A		65.	B
16.	B		66.	A
17.	A		67.	B
18.	B		68.	A
19.	C		69.	C
20.	A		70.	D
21.	A		71.	B
22.	A		72.	C
23.	A		73.	B
24.	A		74.	D
25.	C		75.	D
26.	B		76.	D
27.	A		77.	A
28.	D		78.	B
29.	A		79.	A
30.	A		80.	D
31.	D		81.	A
32.	C		82.	C
33.	B		83.	C
34.	A		84.	B
35.	D		85.	D
36.	A		86.	A
37.	B		87.	B
38.	B		88.	B
39.	A		89.	A
40.	C		90.	A
41.	A		91.	B
42.	A		92.	A
43.	C		93.	C
44.	A		94.	D
45.	D		95.	A
46.	B		96.	A
47.	A		97.	B
48.	D		98.	A
49.	C		99.	C
50.	A		100.	B

CPSIA information can be obtained at www.ICGtesting.com
Printed in the USA
BVOW10s2217100615

404164BV00005B/10/P